my revision notes

Edexcel GCSE (9–1) History

MEDICINE IN BRITAIN

c.1250–PRESENT & THE BRITISH SECTOR OF THE WESTERN FRONT, 1914–18

Sam Slater

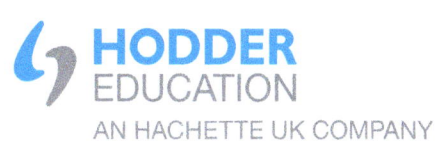

In order to ensure this resource offers high-quality support for the associated Pearson qualification, it has been through a review process by the awarding body. This process confirms that this resource fully covers the teaching and learning content of the specification or part of a specification at which it is aimed. It also confirms that it demonstrates an appropriate balance between the development of subject skills, knowledge and understanding, in addition to preparation for assessment.

Endorsement does not cover any guidance on assessment activities or processes (e.g. practice questions or advice on how to answer assessment questions), included in the resource nor does it prescribe any particular approach to the teaching or delivery of a related course.

While the publishers have made every attempt to ensure that advice on the qualification and its assessment is accurate, the official specification and associated assessment guidance materials are the only authoritative source of information and should always be referred to for definitive guidance. Pearson examiners have not contributed to any sections in this resource relevant to examination papers for which they have responsibility. Examiners will not use endorsed resources as a source of material for any assessment set by Pearson. Endorsement of a resource does not mean that the resource is required to achieve this Pearson qualification, nor does it mean that it is the only suitable material available to support the qualification, and any resource lists produced by the awarding body shall include this and other appropriate resources.

The Publishers would like to thank the following for permission to reproduce copyright material.

Photo credits: p35 The Print Collector/HIP/TopFoto; **p37** Granger, NYC/TopFoto; **p42** TopFoto.

Acknowledgements: mark schemes reproduced by kind permission of Pearson Education Ltd

Every effort has been made to trace all copyright holders, but if any have been inadvertently overlooked, the Publishers will be pleased to make the necessary arrangements at the first opportunity.

Although every effort has been made to ensure that website addresses are correct at time of going to press, Hodder Education cannot be held responsible for the content of any website mentioned in this book. It is sometimes possible to find a relocated web page by typing in the address of the home page for a website in the URL window of your browser.

Hachette UK's policy is to use papers that are natural, renewable and recyclable products and made from wood grown in well-managed forests and other controlled sources. The logging and manufacturing processes are expected to conform to the environmental regulations of the country of origin.

Orders: please contact Hachette UK Distribution, Hely Hutchinson Centre, Milton Road, Didcot, Oxfordshire, OX11 7HH. Telephone: +44 (0)1235 827827. Email education@hachette.co.uk Lines are open from 9 a.m. to 5 p.m., Monday to Friday. You can also order through our website: www.hoddereducation.co.uk

The authorised representative in the EEA is Hachette Ireland, 8 Castlecourt Centre, Dublin 15, D15 XTP3, Ireland (email: info@hbgi.ie)

ISBN: 978 1 5104 0321 5

© Sam Slater 2017

First published in 2017 by
Hodder Education
An Hachette UK Company
Carmelite House, 50 Victoria Embankment
London EC4Y 0DZ

www.hoddereducation.co.uk

Impression number   11
Year   2024

All rights reserved. Apart from any use permitted under UK copyright law, no part of this publication may be reproduced or transmitted in any form or by any means, electronic or mechanical, including photocopying and recording, or held within any information storage and retrieval system, without permission in writing from the publisher or under licence from the Copyright Licensing Agency Limited. Further details of such licences (for reprographic reproduction) may be obtained from the Copyright Licensing Agency Limited, www.cla.co.uk

Cover photo © Marc Tielemans/Alamy Stock Photo
Illustrations by Gray Publishing
Produced and typeset in Bembo by Gray Publishing, Tunbridge Wells, Kent
Printed in the UK

A catalogue record for this title is available from the British Library.

How to get the most out of this book

This book will help you revise for the thematic study and historic environment: Medicine in Britain, c.1250–present and the British sector of the Western Front, 1914–18: injuries, treatment and the trenches.

Use the revision planner on pages 2–3 to track your progress, topic by topic. Tick each box when you have:

1 revised and understood each topic
2 completed the activities
3 checked your answers online.

The content in the book is organised into a series of double-page spreads which cover the specification's content. The left-hand page on each spread has the key content for each topic, and the right-hand page has one or two activities to help you with exam skills or to learn the knowledge you need. Answers to these activities can be found online at www.hoddereducation.co.uk/myrevisionnotes. Quick multiple-choice quizzes to test your knowledge of each topic can be found on the website.

At the end of the book is an exam focus section (pages 40–46) which gives you guidance on how to answer each exam question type.

There are a variety of **activities** for you to complete related to the content on the left-hand page. Some are based on **exam-style questions** which aim to consolidate your revision and practise your exam skills. Others are **revision tasks** to make sure that you have understood every topic and to help you record the key information about each topic.

Tick to track your progress as you revise each element of the key content.

Content for each topic is on the left-hand page.

Key terms, **Key individuals** and **Key factors** are highlighted in the section colour the first time they appear, with an explanation nearby in the margin. As you work through this book, highlight other key ideas and add your own notes. Make this *your* book.

Shorter **revision tasks** help you remember key points of content.

Throughout the book there are **exam tips** that remind you of key points that will help you in the exam.

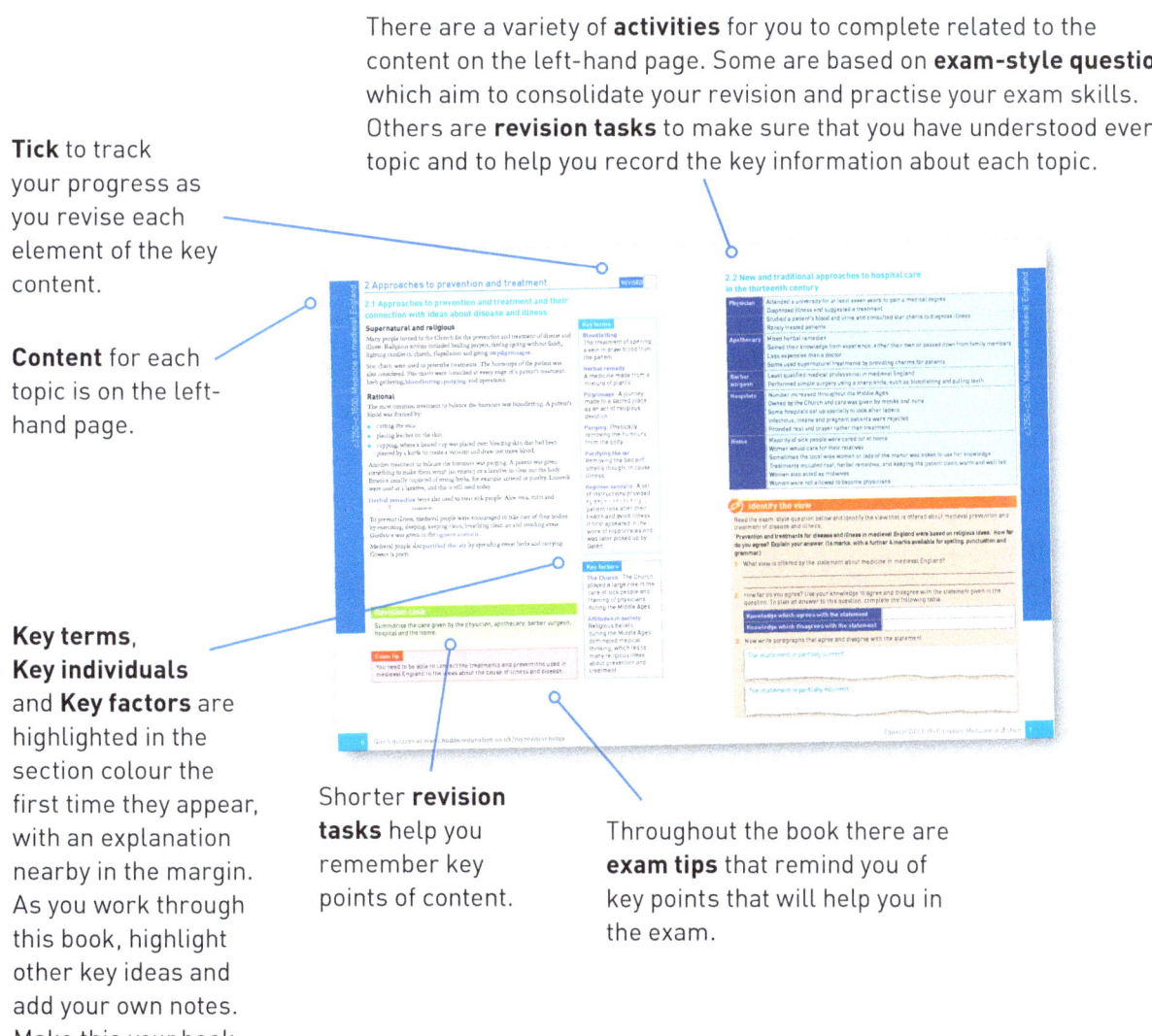

Edexcel GCSE (9–1) History Medicine in Britain

Contents and revision planner

Part 1: Medicine in Britain, c.1250–present

REVISED

- 4 **An overview of medicine from c.1250**
- 5 **The role of factors**

c.1250–c.1500: Medicine in medieval England

1 Ideas about the cause of disease and illness
- 6 1.1 Supernatural and religious explanations
- 6 1.2 Rational explanations

2 Approaches to prevention and treatment
- 8 2.1 Approaches to prevention and treatment and their connection with ideas about disease and illness
- 8 2.2 New and traditional approaches to hospital care in the thirteenth century

3 Case study
- 10 3.1 Dealing with the Black Death, 1348–49

c.1500–c.1700: The Medical Renaissance in England

1 Ideas about the cause of disease and illness
- 12 1.1 Continuity in explanations of the cause of disease and illness
- 12 1.2 Changes in explanations of the cause of disease and illness

2 Approaches to prevention and treatment 1
- 14 2.1 Continuity in approaches to prevention, treatment and care
- 14 2.2 Change in approaches to prevention, treatment and care
- 14 2.3 Dealing with the Great Plague in London in 1665

3 Approaches to prevention and treatment 2
- 16 3.1 Changes in care and treatment
- 16 3.2 William Harvey and the discovery of the circulation of the blood

c.1700–c.1900: Medicine in eighteenth- and nineteenth-century Britain

1 Ideas about the cause of disease and illness
- 18 1.1 Continuity and changes in explanations of the cause of disease and illness
- 18 1.2 The influence of Pasteur's Germ Theory
- 18 1.3 Koch's work on microbes

2 Approaches to prevention and treatment 1
- 20 2.1 The extent of change in care and treatment
- 20 2.2 New approaches to prevention: vaccination

3 Approaches to prevention and treatment 2
- 22   3.1 New approaches to prevention: fighting cholera
- 22   3.2 New approaches to prevention: Public Health Acts

c.1900–present: Medicine in modern Britain

1 Ideas about the cause of disease and illness
- 24   1.1 The influence of genetic factors on health
- 24   1.2 The influence of lifestyle factors on health
- 25   1.3 Improvements in diagnosis

2 Approaches to prevention and treatment 1
- 26   2.1 Advances in medicines
- 26   2.2 Fleming, Florey and Chain's development of penicillin
- 26   2.3 High-tech medical and surgical treatment

3 Approaches to prevention and treatment 2
- 28   3.1 Change in care and treatment
- 28   3.2 New approaches to prevention
- 28   3.3 The fight against lung cancer in the twenty-first century

Part 2: The British sector of the Western Front, 1914–18: injuries, treatment and the trenches
- 30   1   The context of the British sector of the Western Front
- 32   2   Conditions requiring medical treatment on the Western Front
- 34   3   Helping the wounded on the Western Front
- 36   4   The impact of the Western Front on medicine and surgery 1
- 38   5   The impact of the Western Front on medicine and surgery 2

Exam focus
- Question 1: Key features
- Question 2: Source analysis
- Question 2(a): Utility
- Question 2(b): Framing a historical question
- Question 3: Similarity or difference
- Question 4: Causation
- Question 5 and 6: A judgement about change, continuity and significance

Part 1 Medicine in Britain, c.1250–present

An overview of medicine from c.1250

REVISED

Medicine in Britain is a development study. It is important that you have a secure chronological understanding of the content – what happened, and when. You also need to be able to identify change and continuity in the understanding of the cause of disease and illness, and in the methods of prevention and treatment.

Revision task

Create your own medicine timeline by copying this timeline. Make it bigger. You could use a roll of lining paper. As you work through this book, add key events, individuals and discoveries.

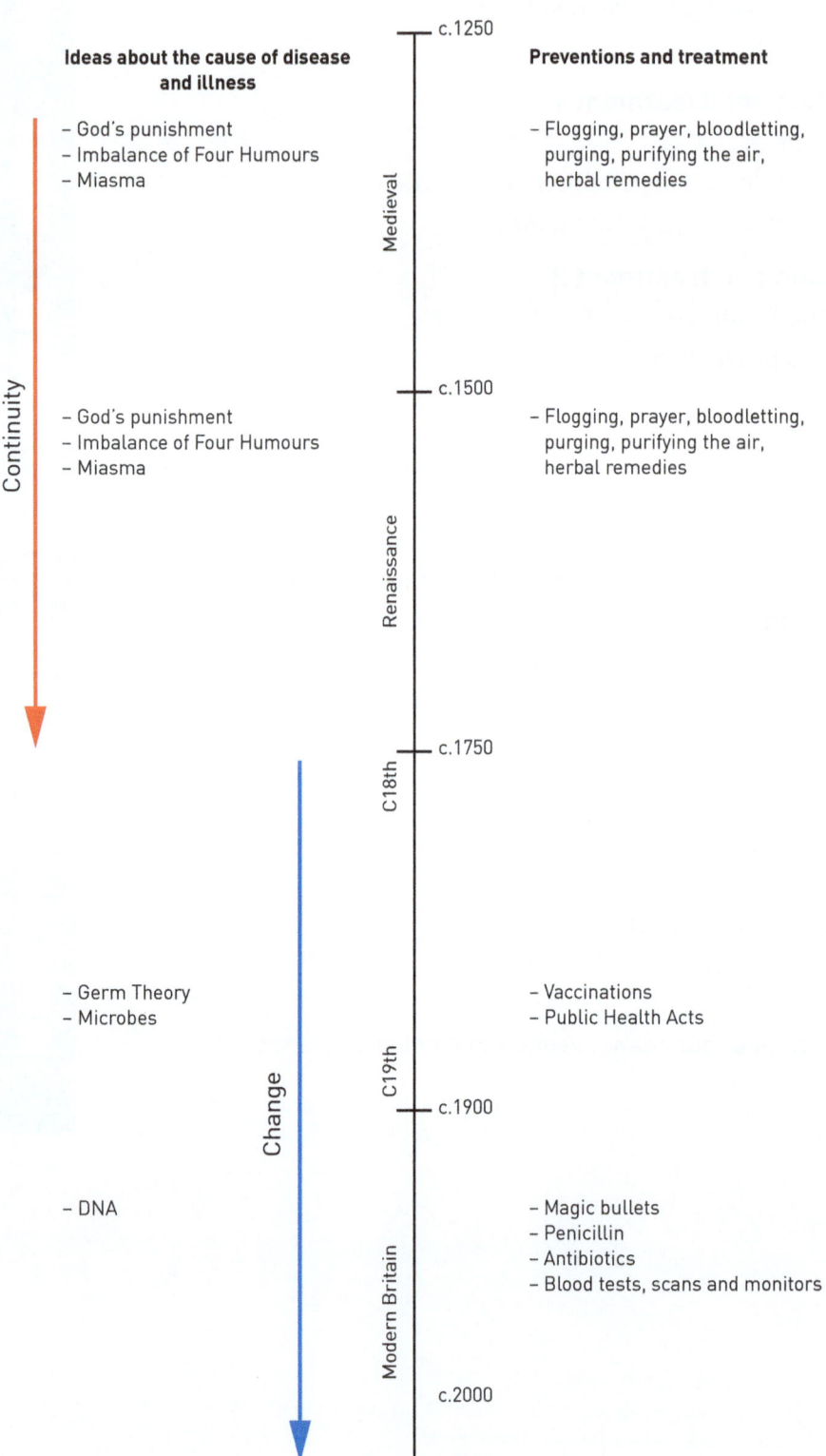

Exam tip

You need to be aware of what changed and continued in medicine from c.1250 to the present day. Look for patterns, trends and turning points.

Quick quizzes at www.hoddereducation.co.uk/myrevisionnotes

The role of factors

Factors are things that influenced medicine in the following ways:

- They helped to cause change: for example, the factor science and technology led to Pasteur discovering germs after experimenting with milk in 1860.
- They helped to prevent change: for example, the factor of the Church hindered any advance in medical knowledge during the medieval period because the Church protected the ideas of Galen and did not allow them to be challenged.

The main factors that you could be asked about in your exam are shown in the diagram below, with an explanation of what they mean.

REVISED

Revision task

Create a table of the factors in each time period that led to a change in medical understanding of the cause of disease and illness and new preventions and treatment. Repeat this for the care provided within the community.

Individuals
Individuals changed medicine, mostly scientists and doctors who made significant medical discoveries.

The institution of the Church
The Church and its ideas influenced medicine throughout the period, sometimes preventing new ideas.

Five key factors which encouraged or inhibited change

Science and technology
New discoveries (science) and inventions (technology) usually encouraged change. Some of these were not directly linked to medicine, e.g. the printing press, but they still had an impact.

Attitudes in society
Beliefs among the population that encouraged and inhibited change, particularly those connected to new discoveries.

The institution of the government
The group of people who governed the country and enforced change in prevention and treatment.

Exam tip

You need to be aware of what and how each factor contributed to medical developments during each time period. Look at what factors caused change and continuity. Look for patterns and trends.

c.1250–c.1500: Medicine in medieval England

The Church and religious beliefs had a great influence over medicine during this period, leading to a continuation of ideas about cause, preventions and treatments.

1 Ideas about the cause of disease and illness

REVISED

Medieval England was a religious society. The majority of people followed the teachings of the Catholic Church and attended services regularly. The cause of disease and illness was unknown due to the lack of scientific knowledge. The majority of people in medieval England could not read or write and would learn from what they heard in church about the causes of illness and disease. The Church controlled education and the universities, where **physicians** were trained.

1.1 Supernatural and religious explanations

Supernatural explanation	Religious explanations
Astrology, the alignment of the planets and stars, was used when diagnosing illness	The Church taught that people's sins were to blame for their illnesses and that illness and disease were sent as a punishment from God
Star charts (map of the night sky) would be consulted by looking at when a patient was born and when they fell ill to help provide a **diagnosis** of what was wrong with them	When people recovered, the Church declared that this was thanks to the patient's prayers
	The Church also taught that disease was sent by God to cleanse the soul of sin or to test your faith

1.2 Rational explanations

Theory of the Four Humours	Miasma Theory
The Theory of the Four Humours was developed in Ancient Greece by **Hippocrates**	A **miasma** was bad air that was believed to be harmful
It continued to influence medical ideas in medieval England	In medieval England it was believed that bad air and smells contained poisonous fumes that caused disease and illness
This theory suggested that the body was made up of four liquids (humours) – blood, phlegm, black and yellow bile – and an imbalance of these substances caused illness and disease	Medieval beliefs suggested that any rotting matter could transmit disease
It was believed that an equal balance of the humours led to good health	

The influence of Hippocrates and Galen

Galen, a physician in Ancient Rome, extended the Theory of the Four Humours by suggesting that the humours should be rebalanced by using the Theory of Opposites. He suggested that too much phlegm, for example, was caused by cold and the 'opposite' should be used, such as hot chillies and peppers to rebalance the humour. Galen also believed in the idea of the soul, which fitted with the teachings of the Church. This led to the Church promoting the ideas of Galen, and doctors widely using the Theory of the Four Humours, throughout the period c.1250–c.1500.

Key terms

Diagnosis Identifying the nature of an illness after considering the different symptoms

Miasma Smells from decomposing material were believed to cause disease

Physician A person qualified to practise medicine

Rational An idea based on logic

Supernatural Ideas unable to be explained by science or the laws of nature

Key individuals

Galen A doctor in Ancient Rome. Galen had his ideas recorded in more than 350 books

Hippocrates A leading physician from Ancient Greece. Hippocrates created the Theory of the Four Humours after carefully observing and recording the symptoms of his patients

Key factors

The Church It was very influential during the Middle Ages and religion was used to explain the causes of illness.

Attitudes in society Religious beliefs in the Middle Ages dominated medical thinking. Galen's ideas continued as the Church accepted them.

Memory map

Create a memory map to show the different ideas that people in medieval England had about the cause of disease. Add some key words from the information on page 6 and your own knowledge to the diagram below. Use two different colours to show whether they are religious and supernatural explanations or rational explanations. To help you remember the information, you could add small drawings.

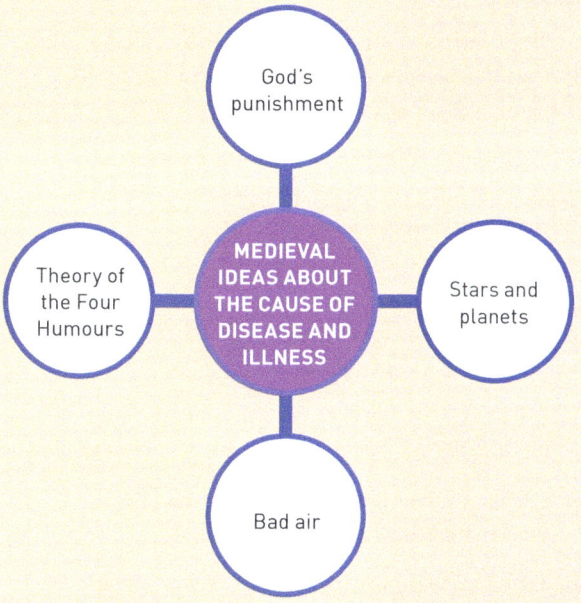

Eliminate irrelevance

Here is an exam-style question:

Explain why there was continuity in ideas about the cause of disease during the period c.1250–c.1500. (12 marks)

> You may use the following in your answer:
> - The Church
> - Galen
>
> You **must** also use information of your own.

Below is a paragraph which is part of an answer to the question above. Some parts of the answer are not relevant to the question. Identify these and draw a line through the information that is irrelevant, justifying your deletions in the margin.

> In medieval England there were religious and supernatural explanations for the cause of illness. The Church was very powerful and controlled education throughout the period, which led to the continuity of ideas. The Church taught that God was responsible for illness and disease. The Church taught that God sent disease as a punishment for sin or to cleanse the soul. As a result of this, many people would also turn to the Church for treatments and preventions. Religious believers would attend church and pray, pay for a special mass to be said to remove their sin and also fast. Some believers would go on a pilgrimage and during the Black Death in 1348 flagellants across Europe would whip themselves to show God how sorry they were for their sins and to show that they did not need to be punished with the disease. These beliefs continued throughout the period c.1250–c.1500 because the Church remained in control of education and continued to teach these ideas. Due to the power that the Church held in society, there was no challenge of the religious explanations, treatments and preventions for disease and illness.

2 Approaches to prevention and treatment

2.1 Approaches to prevention and treatment and their connection with ideas about disease and illness

Supernatural and religious

Many people turned to the Church for the prevention and treatment of disease and illness. Religious actions included healing prayers, fasting (going without food), lighting candles in church, flagellation and going on **pilgrimages**.

Star charts were used to prescribe treatments. The horoscope of the patient was also considered. Star charts were consulted at every stage of a patient's treatment: herb gathering, **bloodletting**, **purging** and operations.

Rational

The most common treatment to balance the humours was bloodletting. A patient's blood was drained by:

- cutting the vein
- placing leeches on the skin
- cupping, where a heated cup was placed over bleeding skin that had been pierced by a knife to create a vacuum and draw out more blood.

Another treatment to balance the humours was purging. A patient was given something to make them vomit (an emetic) or a laxative to clear out the body. Emetics usually consisted of strong herbs, for example aniseed or parsley. Linseeds were used as a laxative, and this is still used today.

Herbal remedies were also used to treat sick people. Aloe vera, mint and camomile were common.

To prevent illness, medieval people were encouraged to take care of their bodies by exercising, sleeping, keeping clean, breathing clean air and avoiding stress. Guidance was given in the *regimen sanitatis*.

Medieval people also **purified the air** by spreading sweet herbs and carrying flowers (a posy).

> **Key terms**
>
> **Bloodletting** The treatment of opening a vein to draw blood from the patient
>
> **Herbal remedy** A medicine made from a mixture of plants
>
> **Pilgrimage** A journey made to a sacred place as an act of religious devotion
>
> **Purging** Physically removing the humours from the body
>
> **Purifying the air** Removing the bad air/smells thought to cause illness
>
> *Regimen sanitatis* A set of instructions provided by physicians to help a patient look after their health and avoid illness. It first appeared in the work of Hippocrates and was later picked up by Galen

> **Key factors**
>
> **The Church** The Church played a large role in the care of sick people and training of physicians during the Middle Ages.
>
> **Attitudes in society** Religious beliefs during the Middle Ages dominated medical thinking, which led to many religious ideas about prevention and treatment.

> **Revision task**
>
> Summarise the care given by the physician, apothecary, barber surgeon, hospital and the home.

> **Exam tip**
>
> You need to be able to connect the treatments and preventions used in medieval England to the ideas about the cause of illness and disease.

2.2 New and traditional approaches to hospital care in the thirteenth century

Physician	Attended a university for at least seven years to gain a medical degree
	Diagnosed illness and suggested a treatment
	Studied a patient's blood and urine and consulted star charts to diagnose illness
	Rarely treated patients
Apothecary	Mixed herbal remedies
	Gained their knowledge from experience; either their own or passed down from family members
	Less expensive than a doctor
	Some used supernatural treatments by providing charms for patients
Barber surgeon	Least qualified medical professional in medieval England
	Performed simple surgery using a sharp knife, such as bloodletting and pulling teeth
Hospitals	Number increased throughout the Middle Ages
	Owned by the Church and care was given by monks and nuns
	Some hospitals set up specially to look after lepers
	Infectious, insane and pregnant patients were rejected
	Provided rest and prayer rather than treatment
Home	Majority of sick people were cared for at home
	Women would care for their relatives
	Sometimes the local wise woman or lady of the manor was asked to use her knowledge
	Treatments included rest, herbal remedies, and keeping the patient clean, warm and well fed
	Women also acted as midwives
	Women were not allowed to become physicians

Identify the view

Read the exam-style question below and identify the view that is offered about medieval prevention and treatment of disease and illness.

'Prevention and treatments for disease and illness in medieval England were based on religious ideas.' How far do you agree? Explain your answer. (16 marks, with a further 4 marks available for spelling, punctuation and grammar.)

1. What view is offered by the statement about medicine in medieval England?

2. How far do you agree? Use your knowledge to agree and disagree with the statement given in the question. To plan an answer to this question, complete the following table.

Knowledge which agrees with the statement	
Knowledge which disagrees with the statement	

3. Now write paragraphs that agree and disagree with the statement.

The statement is partially correct …

The statement is partially incorrect …

3 Case study: Dealing with the Black Death, 1348–49

REVISED

The Black Death was an outbreak of the **bubonic plague** that first broke out in China and reached England in 1348. It is believed to have killed 40 per cent of the population of England. It was unlikely a victim would survive the disease once they caught it; they would die within three to five days. We know little about the treatments because its victims died so quickly.

Beliefs about the causes

Beliefs about the causes related to medieval views about the world, including:
- God had sent the disease as a punishment for sins.
- An unusual alignment of the planets Mars, Jupiter and Saturn in 1345.
- An imbalance of the four humours (see page 6) or the existence of evil humours within the body.
- Bad air (miasma) which had corrupted the body's humours. This poisonous air was believed to have been released from a volcano or an earthquake.

Approaches to treatment

Treatments for the Black Death related to the ideas about its causes:
- People prayed, confessed sins, donated and asked God for forgiveness.
- Holy charms were worn to show one's religious beliefs.
- Bleeding, purging and treatments based on Galen's Theory of Opposites (see page 6) were used to rebalance the four humours.
- A victim would sniff strong herbs, such as myrrh, in order to replace the bad air in their body.
- Many victims would light fires to remove the bad air and replace it with the smoke and fumes from the fire.
- Because some victims survived once the pus was released, victims would lance the buboes in the hope that this would cure them of the disease.

Attempts to prevent its spread

Ways to prevent the Black Death from spreading centred around religion, keeping the streets clean to prevent bad air and isolating its victims.
- Many would pray to God in the hope of avoiding punishment.
- The king and bishops ordered processions in every church at least once a day.
- People went on pilgrimages and made sacrifices to God, such as fasting.
- **Flagellants** whipped themselves to ask for God's forgiveness.
- People carried posies of sweet-smelling herbs and flowers.
- Rakers cleared animal dung from the streets to stop creating bad air.
- Fines for throwing litter were increased to keep the streets cleaner.
- To reduce the waste on the streets, butchers had to use segregated areas to butcher animals or face punishment.
- Ringing bells and birds were used to keep the air moving.
- New quarantine laws were issued to prevent the movement of people. Those new to an area had to remain isolated for 40 days, to ensure they were not infected.
- The authorities **quarantined** houses of victims.

Key terms

Bubonic plague A contagious and fatal epidemic disease caused by bacteria and characterised by chills, fever, vomiting and buboes

Flagellants Religious believers who whipped themselves to show God that they repented their sins and to ask for his forgiveness to avoid the plague

Quarantine Separating sick people to stop the spread of disease. Those with the disease were isolated in the quarantined area

Exam tip

You need to be able to explain the link between what people did to treat and prevent the Black Death and the medieval beliefs that existed about the cause of disease.

Organising knowledge

Use the information on page 10 to complete the table below to show the links between cause, treatment and prevention of the Black Death.

Black Death	Religion	Rational	Supernatural
Beliefs about cause			
Treatment			
Prevention			

Analysing factors

You need to understand the role that factors had on the medieval ideas about the cause of disease and the treatments and preventions that they used. Make a copy of the concentric circles. Rank order the factors in the box that explain the ideas that existed about cause, treatment and prevention, beginning with the most important in the middle to the least important on the outside. Explain your decisions by annotating the diagram.

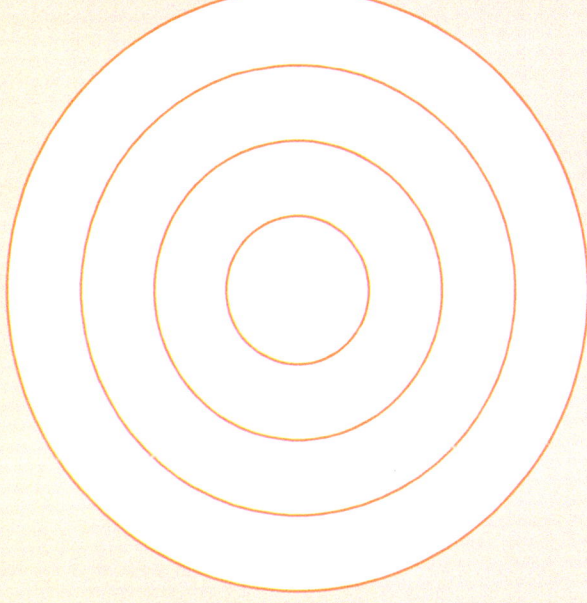

For example, if you believe that the religious ideas about cause, treatment and prevention were the most influential, write 'The Church' in the centre circle. You can then annotate this with details of the religious ideas, such as it was believed that God sent the Black Death as a punishment for sins.

FACTORS
- government
- individuals
- attitudes in society
- the Church
- science and technology.

For a reminder about each factor see page 5.

c.1250–c.1500: Medicine in medieval England

Edexcel GCSE (9–1) History Medicine in Britain

c.1500–c.1700: The Medical Renaissance in England

Ideas about the causes of disease and illness were starting to change during the Renaissance. However, this led to very little change in methods of prevention and treatment. The Renaissance did see the introduction of science and technology improving medicine.

1 Ideas about the cause of disease and illness

REVISED

During the Medical Renaissance new ideas began to influence medicine and slowly replace old beliefs. As Protestantism spread across Europe, the Catholic Church was less able to promote its beliefs and control medicine. As a more secular society developed, scientific ideas were discovered both in medicine, and beyond.

1.1 Continuity in explanations of the cause of disease and illness

- Miasma Theory (see page 6): this idea continued and became more widespread during epidemics.
- The influence of the Church: during epidemics, such as the Great Plague, religious causes were still influential.
- Supernatural: from 1500, astrology was less popular, but during epidemics people continued to wear charms as protection from evil spirits.

1.2 Changes in explanations of the cause of disease and illness

The practice of medicine did not change much during this time, but the ideas about cause were starting to change:

- The decline in influence of the Church: most now believed that God did not send disease.
- The Theory of the Four Humours: this had been discredited and was not believed by physicians by the end of the seventeenth century. However, because patients understood it, the theory continued to be used to diagnose illness until this time.
- Urine analysis: physicians now understood that urine was not linked to ill health and no longer used it to diagnose illness.

By the end of the Renaissance, there was a move away from old ideas about medicine, but they had not been replaced.

Animalcules

A new idea that little animals were the cause of illness developed after they could be seen by newly invented, more powerful microscopes. These images were not very clear.

The work of Thomas Sydenham

Thomas Sydenham was important in moving medicine away from the ideas of Hippocrates and Galen. Sydenham believed in closely observing the symptoms of a patient, noting these down in detailed descriptions and then looking for remedies to treat the disease, rather than relying on medical books.

> **Key terms**
>
> **Epidemic** A widespread occurrence of an infectious disease in a community at a particular time
>
> **Printing press** A machine for reproducing text and pictures
>
> **Protestantism** The practice of the Protestant Church
>
> **Renaissance** A revival of ideas from 1500 to 1700
>
> **Secular** Not connected with religious or spiritual matters

> **Key individual**
>
> **Thomas Sydenham** A well-respected doctor in London during the 1660s and 1670s. He was given the nickname of the 'English Hippocrates' because, like the Greek doctor, he placed great importance on observing a patient. His book *Observationes Medicae* was used for two centuries

The influence of the printing press

In the fifteenth century, the first printing press was invented. It enabled medical information to spread further and more quickly; and contributed to the decline in influence of the Church. Now physicians were able to publish books that criticised Galen.

The Royal Society

The Royal Society was founded in London in 1660 to discuss new ideas in astronomy, medicine and science. It was important in the development of new medical ideas because it made it possible for scientists and physicians to study one another's work. The Royal Society also sponsored scientists and assisted them with the publication of their ideas.

> **Key factor**
>
> **Science and technology**
> Science began to play a significant role in medicine during the Renaissance. Physicians and doctors started to question the old ideas and look to science for new explanations for the cause of disease and illness. New technology was developed that assisted the development of medicine; the printing press and microscopes.

Organising knowledge

Use the information on page 12 to complete the table below to show the old and new ideas that existed during the Renaissance in England about the cause of disease and illness.

| Ideas about the cause of disease and illness during the medical Renaissance in England ||
New ideas	Old ideas

Making comparisons

Look at the exam-style question below and the two answers. Which answer is better for comparing the key features of medical understanding? Why?

Explain one way in which ideas about the causes of disease were similar in the fourteenth and seventeenth centuries. (4 marks)

> **ANSWER 1**
>
> Ideas about the causes of disease in the fourteenth and seventeenth centuries were similar because at both times illness was believed to have been caused by bad air.

> **ANSWER 2**
>
> In the fourteenth and seventeenth centuries disease was believed to have a rational cause, for example bad air (miasma). During the Great Plague, like the Black Death, people believed that bad air (miasma) was caused by rotting waste and a movement of the planets. They believed that this led to an imbalance of the four humours and so disease in the form of the plague.

2 Approaches to prevention and treatment 1

2.1 Continuity in approaches to prevention, treatment and care

Many of the preventions and treatments used during medieval England continued throughout the Renaissance because there was little change in the ideas about the cause of illness. These included:

- bloodletting, purging and sweating
- herbal remedies
- the practice of *regimen sanitatis* (see page 8)
- the removal of bad air
- treatment of sick people by apothecaries and surgeons for those who could not afford a physician
- women cared for sick people who did not go to hospital.

2.2 Changes in approaches to prevention, treatment and care

The move towards scientific thinking also led to new preventions and treatments:

- People started to believe in **transference**.
- People began to look for chemical cures for diseases rather than relying on herbs and bloodletting.
- Ideas that the weather conditions were the cause of disease became more popular and so people would relocate to avoid a disease.
- Renaissance hospitals began to treat people with wounds and curable diseases such as fevers.
- Hospitals that specialised in one particular disease were new in this period. These became known as pest houses, plague houses or poxhouses.

2.3 Dealing with the Great Plague in London in 1665

The plague returned to England throughout the seventeenth century. The Great Plague was the last major epidemic of the plague to hit England.

Key terms

Pomander A ball that contained perfumed substances

Transference Belief that an illness or disease could be transferred to something else. For example, people believed that if you rubbed an object on a boil the disease would transfer from the person to the object

Revision task

Summarise the continuity in the prevention and treatment of disease and illness in the period c.1250–c.1700. Try to make this visual by creating a mind map.

Exam tip

You need to know the similarities and differences between the preventions and treatments during the Great Plague in 1665 those used during the Black Death in 1348.

Idea about cause	Prevention and treatment
Astrology: an unusual alignment of the planets	Prayers were recited
	Plague victims were quarantined for 28 days and the door was painted with a cross alongside the words 'Lord have mercy upon us'
Punishment from God to cleanse man of his sins	People were encouraged to carry a **pomander** to drive away the bad air
	Fasting took place and some changed their diet to include a lot of garlic
An imbalance of the four humours	Plague doctors treated patients wearing a birdlike mask (because birds were believed to attract disease away from the patient), with sweet-smelling herbs inside to ward off miasma
Miasma: bad air caused by foul-smelling rubbish	Smoking tobacco to ward off miasma
Person to person by touch	Local authorities tried to prevent the plague from spreading by: • banning public meetings, funerals and fairs • closing theatres • sweeping streets clean • burning barrels of tar and sweet-smelling herbs to ward off miasma • killing cats and dogs • appointing searchers to monitor the spread of the disease and clear victims' bodies from towns

Organising knowledge

Study the Black Death in 1348 (page 10) and the Great Plague in 1665 (page 14). Complete the table below to show the similarities and differences between these two outbreaks.

Similarities	Differences
Ideas about the cause:	Ideas about the cause:
Preventions and treatments:	Preventions and treatments:

You're the examiner

Below is an exam-style question.

Explain why there was continuity in the way disease and illness were prevented and treated in the period c.1250–c.1700. (12 marks)

You may use the following information in your answer:
- Great Plague
- Attitudes in society

1. Below are a mark scheme and a paragraph which is part of an answer to the question. Read the paragraph and the mark scheme. Decide which level you would award the paragraph. Write the level below, along with a justification for your choice.

   Remember that for the higher levels you must:
   - explain three reasons
   - focus explicitly on the question
   - support reasons with precise details.

Mark scheme	
Level	
1	A simple or generalised answer is given, lacking development and organisation
2	An explanation is given, showing limited analysis and with only an implicit link to the question
3	An explanation is given, showing some analysis, which is mainly directed at the focus of the question
4	An analytical explanation is given which is directed consistently at the focus of the question

STUDENT ANSWER

People tried to prevent catching the Great Plague by placing those who had the disease in quarantine for 28 days, by carrying a pomander to drive away the miasma because they believed it was caused by the bad air, and by eating a diet heavy with garlic. Some healers advised smoking tobacco to also ward off the miasma. Local government also took action by banning public meetings and fairs, and closing theatres. Fires were lit and barrels of tar were burned. These actions took place because the local government wanted to prevent the spread of the disease by contagion and miasma. Here we can see a similarity with the Black Death during the Middle Ages as this epidemic was also believed to have been spread by bad air and contagion.

Level [ ]   Reason _____

2. Now suggest what the student has to do to achieve a higher level.

3. Try and rewrite this paragraph at a higher level.
4. Now try and write the rest of the answer to the question.

3 Approaches to prevention and treatment 2

3.1 Changes in care and treatment

The new approach to medicine and knowledge developed during the Renaissance led to a change in medical training and care of sick people.

Improvements in medical training

Apothecaries and surgeons were better educated between 1500 and 1700:

- Wars were being fought with new technology, which led to new wounds that required more surgery.
- The increase in available chemicals led to new ingredients being available for apothecaries.

Physicians continued to train at universities with little change. Due to the decline in power of the Church, **dissection** was legalised but it was difficult to get a supply of fresh corpses to work on. This meant that physicians continued to train from books, such as those of Galen. Training did advance as physicians were inspired to challenge the old teachings and investigate for themselves (see below, Vesalius and Harvey). The printing press made books more widely available for physicians to study.

The influence in England of the work of Vesalius

In 1543, **Vesalius** published his most famous book, *On the Fabric of the Human Body*. Vesalius had been able to dissect a large number of executed criminals.

Learning of Vesalius	Impact of Vesalius
Vesalius found around 300 mistakes in the anatomical work of Galen, which included: • the human lower jaw has one bone, not two • the human breastbone has three parts, not seven • men do not have one fewer pair of ribs than women • the human liver does not have five separate lobes	Anatomy became central to the study of medicine, and doctors were encouraged to carry out dissections for themselves
	Vesalius' work was heavily copied and appeared in other medical texts
Vesalius corrected these mistakes and encouraged other doctors to base their work on dissection rather than old books. Vesalius explained these mistakes by pointing out that Galen had dissected animals, rather than humans	His work inspired other anatomists. After Vesalius' death, Fabricius went on to discover valves in human veins and shared his discovery with William Harvey
	Vesalius caused a lot of controversy because he had challenged the ideas of Galen. This angered traditional physicians who argued that the human body had not changed since the ideas of Galen

> **Key terms**
>
> **Anatomy** The branch of science concerned with the bodily structure of humans
>
> **Dissection** Cutting up a body to study its internal parts

> **Key individuals**
>
> **William Harvey** Studied medicine at Cambridge and then at the famous medical school in Padua. In 1615, he became a lecturer in anatomy at the College of Physicians before becoming a doctor to King James I
>
> **Andreas Vesalius** The most famous anatomist of this period. He was a lecturer in surgery at the University of Padua and had a deep interest in the human body

> **Key factor**
>
> **Individuals** The work of individuals became important during the medical Renaissance in England. What they discovered about the human body is important, but also the influence that they had.

> **Revision task**
>
> Summarise in no more than ten words the changes in medical training and treatment as a result of the work of Vesalius and Harvey.

3.2 William Harvey and the discovery of the circulation of the blood

Harvey had a keen interest in dissection and observing the human body to improve his knowledge of human anatomy.

Discovery of the circulation of the blood	Impact of Harvey
Harvey's research involved dissecting human corpses and cutting open cold-blooded animals because they had a slower heartbeat and this enabled their blood to be observed while they were still alive	Harvey's theory encouraged other scientists to experiment on actual bodies
Harvey's research proved that arteries and veins were linked together in one system	However, his discovery had little practical use in medical treatment and led to very little change
Harvey's theory was that blood must pass from arteries to veins through tiny passages invisible to the naked eye. Today we know these to be capillaries	Some openly criticised Harvey because he did not have a powerful enough microscope to prove that capillaries existed. He was said to be mad
Harvey corrected Galen and showed that only the veins carried blood and that the heart acted as a pump	

Support or challenge

Below is an exam-style question which asks how far you agree with a specific statement. Below this are a series of general statements which are relevant to the question. Using your own knowledge and the information throughout this key topic, decide whether these statements support or challenge the statement in the question and tick the appropriate box.

'Individuals had the most significant impact on medical training between c.1500 and c.1700.' How far do you agree? Explain your answer. (16 marks, with a further 4 marks available for spelling, punctuation and grammar.)

> You may use the following in your answer:
> - Vesalius
> - The Royal Society
>
> You **must** also use some information of your own.

Statement	Support	Challenge
More powerful microscopes were being developed and, in 1683, one allowed for the observation of tiny 'animalcules'		
The Royal Society first met in 1660 to share scientific knowledge and encourage new ideas		
The Theory of the Four Humours was starting to be rejected by physicians		
Doctors and anatomists were starting to observe the human body themselves rather than relying on old books		
Thomas Sydenham encouraged doctors to observe their patients and note down their symptoms		
The newly developed printing press allowed for medical information to be spread quickly and accurately		
Vesalius dissected human corpses and proved around 300 ideas of Galen incorrect		
Harvey discovered that blood circulated around the body and that the heart acted as a pump		
Without a microscope, Harvey was unable to prove that capillaries existed and so many physicians ignored his ideas		

Once you have completed this table, write an answer to this question.

c.1700–c.1900: Medicine in eighteenth- and nineteenth-century Britain

From 1700, the Church began to lose its influence over disease and illness as there was a focus on scientific explanations. This period saw the growth of cities, which brought threatening diseases such as smallpox, tuberculosis and typhus.

1 Ideas about the cause of disease and illness

REVISED

Intellectual movements such as the **Enlightenment** encouraged others to think for themselves to find answers – including about disease and illness.

1.1 Continuity and changes in explanations of the cause of disease and illness

Ideas about the cause of disease had not changed by the eighteenth century and people still believed in the Theory of the Four Humours and miasma, but this theory was losing popularity. Scientific thinking led to a change in medical understanding at the end of this period when the **Germ Theory** was developed.

Spontaneous generation theory

Microscopes had improved so that scientists could see **microbes** on decaying matter. This led some scientists to develop the theory of spontaneous generation in the early eighteenth century. They argued that the microbes were a product of the decay, rather than the cause of it, and that they spread by miasma.

1.2 The influence of Pasteur's Germ Theory

In 1861, **Louis Pasteur** published his discovery of the Germ Theory. He proved that germs were causing liquids to decay. This disproved the spontaneous generation theory. This discovery led him to the theory that germs might cause disease in the human body.

Impact

- Little immediate impact on medicine because doctors and surgeons could not see Pasteur's microbes.
- Some impact on the work of Joseph Lister, who linked the Germ Theory to infection in his patients (see page 20). Unfortunately, Lister's ideas were doubted as he could not prove his theory. With the presence of microbes in the organs of healthy people, it seemed impossible to some that they could be the cause of disease and illness.
- In the long term, Pasteur's discovery led to changes in preventing disease with vaccinations and the introduction of antiseptic and aseptic surgery.

1.3 Koch's work on microbes

Robert Koch developed the work of Pasteur by successfully identifying the different microbes that caused common individual diseases:

- 1876: Koch discovered the bacteria that caused anthrax.
- 1882: Koch went on to discover the bacteria that caused tuberculosis and typhoid.
- 1883: Koch discovered cholera.
- Koch's co-workers also went on to discover the microbes for diphtheria, pneumonia, meningitis, the plague and tetanus.

Key terms

Enlightenment A European intellectual movement of the late seventeenth and eighteenth centuries that emphasised reason and individualism rather than tradition

Germ Theory The theory that germs cause disease, often by infection through the air

Microbes A living organism that can only be seen with a microscope. Microbes include bacteria

Key individuals

Robert Koch A German doctor who identified specific bacteria that caused disease in humans

Louis Pasteur A French chemist who discovered germs before going on to develop vaccines

Key factors

Attitudes in society The Enlightenment encouraged questioning and new theories about medicine to develop

Science and technology Scientific experiment, microscopes, the swan-neck flask and the Petri dish were all vital instruments in the discovery of germs and development of vaccines

Koch's influence in Britain	
Positive	**Negative**
Koch made it easier to see microbes by developing a dye that would stain them	The discovery of germs and different bacteria alone did not have an impact on medical treatment. It took time for cures and vaccines to be developed
Koch's new method of growing microbes enabled other scientists to study specific diseases	Initially the British government rejected the idea of the Germ Theory. Even when Koch went to Calcutta and proved that cholera was caused by microbes in the drinking water, they ignored this and continued to believe in miasma
Koch's work inspired other scientists to look for the microbes responsible for other diseases	

Revision task

Create a timeline showing the development of the Germ Theory. Include the work of Pasteur and Koch.

Analysing factors

You need to understand the role that factors had on the ideas about cause of disease and illness in the eighteenth and nineteenth centuries. Copy and complete the diagram below. For each factor in the diagram, explain how it led to advances in the understanding of the cause of disease and illness during this period. If a factor contributed in multiple ways, you will want to have more than one explanation.

Once you have completed the diagram, decide which factor you think was the most significant and why.

For a reminder about each factor see page 5.

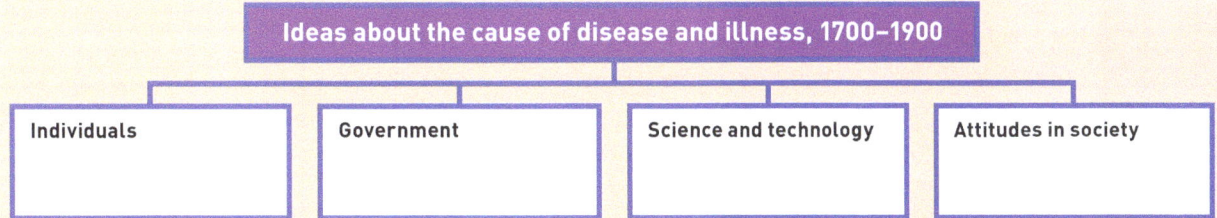

Complete the paragraph

Below are an exam-style question and a paragraph which is part of an answer to this question. The paragraph gives an argument for agreeing with the statement and some historical support but does not go on to develop the explanation.

1. Rewrite the paragraph with extra precise supporting knowledge and a full explanation linking back to the statement.
2. Complete the answer to this question.

'There was complete change in ideas about the cause of disease and illness in the period c.1700–c.1900.' How far do you agree? Explain your answer. (16 marks, with a further 4 marks available for spelling, punctuation and grammar.)

You may use the following information in your answer.
- Germ Theory
- Robert Koch

You **must** also use information of your own.

> There was complete change in the ideas about the cause of disease and illness in the period c.1700–c.1900 because science prevailed and microbes were identified and understood. In 1861, Louis Pasteur discovered and published his Germ Theory. Although Pasteur had only proven that microbes caused decay in liquids, he inspired other scientists to look for a similar cause to explain disease in the human body. Robert Koch followed Pasteur and identified the microbes that caused anthrax, tuberculosis and cholera.

2 Approaches to prevention and treatment 1

2.1 The extent of change in care and treatment

Hospital care	From the eighteenth century more people were treated in a hospital, but this led to less sanitary conditions
	Florence Nightingale trained as a nurse in Germany and Paris before being sent by the government to the Crimea to improve hospitals during the Crimean War
	Nightingale noticed the high death rate among soldiers
	Alongside 38 nurses, Nightingale made changes. The wards were cleaned of any dirt, organisation was improved and patients were given clean bedding and meals. Within six months the death rate fell from 40 per cent to 2 per cent
	Nightingale returned to Britain, campaigning for cleaner hospitals and improved training for nurses. In 1859 she wrote *Notes on Nursing*. In 1860 she set up the Nightingale School for Nurses
	Nightingale also influenced the way hospitals were designed. By 1900 they looked very different; they were built from materials that could easily be cleaned and had separate wards
Surgery	Surgery in the eighteenth century was dangerous. Patients faced the problems of pain, infection and bleeding
	In 1847, **James Simpson** discovered chloroform as an **anaesthetic**
	Doctors had to be careful using chloroform because the dosage had to be carefully controlled. In 1848, Hannah Greener died from an overdose during an operation to have her toenail removed
	Chloroform continued to be used and was given a royal blessing in 1853 when Queen Victoria used it during the birth of her son
	The problem of infection was overcome in 1865 by **Joseph Lister**
	Lister used carbolic acid to clear bacteria from the wounds of patients. This became known as **antiseptic surgery**
	Unfortunately, Lister's ideas faced opposition because the medical profession took time to understand the Germ Theory. The carbolic spray was unpleasant to use; it dried out the skin of surgeons and left an odd smell. From 1890, **aseptic surgery** was performed

2.2 New approaches to prevention: vaccination

Throughout the eighteenth century, smallpox epidemics threatened Britain. Smallpox spread quickly and killed many. There was no understanding about its cause or how to prevent it.

Initially, **inoculation** was used to prevent the spread of smallpox. It was expensive and only available to the rich. Inoculation was dangerous as some patients died from the dose that they were given.

Edward Jenner, a country doctor, observed that milkmaids who had previously suffered from cowpox did not catch smallpox during the epidemics. He believed the two were connected and went on to test his theory in 1796. He gave James Phipps a dose of cowpox and six weeks later infected him with smallpox, but Phipps did not catch it. Jenner repeated his experiment with the same success before publishing his findings.

Key terms

Anaesthetic A chemical used to make a patient unconscious during surgery and so remove pain

Antiseptic surgery The removal of bacteria from an operation. Lister used carbolic acid to wash a surgeon's hands, soak bandages and ligatures, and spray the air directly around the wound

Aseptic surgery Surgery that takes place in a strictly controlled germ-free environment

Inoculation Deliberately infecting oneself with a disease in order to become immune and avoid catching a more severe form later on

Key individuals

Edward Jenner A country doctor who developed the smallpox vaccine following careful observation of milkmaids

Joseph Lister A surgeon who discovered that carbolic acid can be used in the operating theatre to remove germs; known as antiseptic surgery

Florence Nightingale A British nurse in the Crimean War who encouraged better hygiene in hospitals and improved training of nurses to reduce the death rate

James Simpson A surgeon and professor of midwifery who discovered that chloroform can be used as an anaesthetic

It took some time before Jenner's **vaccination** was accepted:

- People opposed the vaccine because Jenner was unable to explain how or why it worked. Pasteur did not publish his Germ Theory until 1861 and so Jenner did not know that bacteria caused disease.
- The idea of infecting someone with an animal disease was considered strange and unacceptable. Many religious believers thought it was against God's law to give people an animal disease.
- Inoculators were against it because their business was under threat.
- The Royal Society refused to publish Jenner's findings because it was thought that his ideas were too revolutionary.
- The Anti-Vaccine Society was set up in 1866 to oppose vaccination. It did this by publishing cartoons to scare people into not trusting the vaccine. One such cartoon showed people who had the vaccine turning into cows.

In 1852, the British government made the smallpox vaccination compulsory, and smallpox was eradicated as a disease in 1980. Jenner's work inspired other scientists, like Pasteur and Koch, to develop vaccines. Pasteur went on to develop vaccines for chicken cholera, anthrax and rabies.

> **Key term**
>
> **Vaccination** The injection into the body of killed or weakened organisms to give the body resistance against disease. The smallpox vaccine was the only one to use a different disease and so is known as a 'dead-end' vaccine

> **Key factor**
>
> **Individuals** The work of Nightingale, Simpson, Lister and Jenner in the nineteenth century was crucial to the prevention and treatment of disease and illness.

Revision task

Summarise the contributions of the following individuals to medical advances during the eighteenth and nineteenth centuries:

- Jenner
- Nightingale
- Simpson
- Lister.

Understand the chronology

The events of the eighteenth and nineteenth centuries that led to a change in the prevention and treatment of disease and illness are very complex. Using pages 18 and 20, place the events listed below in the correct chronological sequence in the timeline.

- A Nightingale set up the Nightingale School of Nurses
- B Koch identified the microbe for anthrax
- C Simpson discovered that chloroform was an anaesthetic
- D Jenner developed the smallpox vaccine
- E Queen Victoria used chloroform during childbirth
- F The British government made the smallpox vaccine compulsory
- G Nightingale wrote *Notes on Nursing*
- H Hannah Greener died from a chloroform overdose
- I Koch identified the microbes for tuberculosis and typhoid
- J Lister used the carbolic spray in the operating theatre
- K Nightingale went to the Crimea to improve hospitals
- L Louis Pasteur published his Germ Theory.

Date	Event
1796	
1847	
1848	
1852	
1853	
1854	
1859	
1860	
1861	
1865	
1876	
1882	

3 Approaches to prevention and treatment 2

3.1 New approaches to prevention: fighting cholera

Cholera was a terrible disease that caused sickness and diarrhoea and was usually fatal. Doctors were unable to treat it because they did not know its cause. It was still believed that disease was caused by miasma and so local councils took steps to clean cities.

In 1854, cholera broke out in Soho, London. People tried to prevent its spread by:

- burning barrels of tar to remove the bad air
- smoking cigars to protect against the bad air
- praying and burning the clothes and bedding of victims.

The 1854 outbreak of cholera prompted **John Snow** to investigate.

- Snow created a spot map to show the deaths from cholera that occurred around Broad Street in the Soho district of London.
- This led Snow to notice a pattern; that the deaths were all connected to the water pump.
- Snow removed the handle of the water pump and prevented people from using it.
- There were no more deaths in the Broad Street area from cholera.
- Snow inspected the well underneath the water pump and found that it was close to a cesspit with a cracked lining. This caused waste to seep into the water and spread cholera.

Snow was able to prove that cholera was spread by dirty water and he presented his evidence to the House of Commons. Snow's evidence and the **Great Stink** led the government to agree to a new sewer system, which was planned by Joseph Bazalgette. By 1865, 1300 miles of sewers had been built in London and this project was completed in 1875.

Snow had no scientific evidence to explain the cause of cholera so many rejected his work. It would need Pasteur's Germ Theory and Koch's identification of the cholera microbe before Snow's theory could be explained.

3.2 New approaches to prevention: Public Health Acts

In the early nineteenth century, the British government had a *laissez-faire* attitude and believed it was not their role to intervene in the health of the people. However, during the century this attitude began to change. This was as a result of a variety of reasons, including:

- Cholera continued to return to Britain and it killed more people. The government listened to Snow (see above) and Pasteur (see page 18).
- In 1842, Edwin Chadwick published his *Report on the Sanitary Conditions of the Labouring Classes*. Chadwick had spent years researching the lives of the poor in Britain's cities. He concluded that people living in the cities had a lower life expectancy because of the filthy conditions. He believed all cities should have a Board of Health that ensured the supply of clean water and disposal of sewage. Initially, there was opposition to Chadwick's ideas due to the need to increase taxes and for the government to get involved in local matters.
- The British government did very little at first, but as more scientific evidence emerged that showed clean water was important for a healthy population, the government took more action.
- 1866–67 saw the last cholera epidemic in Britain and it had a lower death count than previous cholera epidemics.

Key individual

John Snow A surgeon who lived in Soho, London, and became one of the city's leading anaesthetists. He was popular and well respected. During the 1848 cholera epidemic, he observed and concluded that the disease was caused by drinking dirty water

Key terms

Great Stink The hot, dry summer of 1858 caused an awful smell from the exposed sewage on the banks of the River Thames in London. This became known as the Great Stink

Laissez-faire From the French for 'leave alone' and is used to describe the British government's attitude to public health in the early nineteenth century

Key factor

Government During the nineteenth century, the British government became more supportive and increased their role in the prevention of disease and illness. This was as a consequence of the increase in scientific evidence and understanding.

Exam tip

It is important that you can explain government action during this period. Link cause and consequence directly.

The first Public Health Act in 1848	The second Public Health Act in 1875
Cities were encouraged to set up Boards of Health and provide clean water supplies. However, because it was not compulsory many did not	Cities were now forced to improve sanitary conditions by: • providing clean water to stop the spread of disease • disposing of sewage to avoid pollution • building public toilets • employing a public officer of health to monitor conditions and outbreaks of disease • creating street lighting

RAG: Rate the timeline

Below are an exam-style question and a timeline. Read the question, study the timeline and, using three coloured pens, put a red, amber or green star next to the events to show:

Red: events that have **no** relevance to the question

Amber: events that have **some** significance to the question

Green: events that have **direct** relevance to the question

Explain why the government increased its role in preventing disease and illness during the period c.1700–c.1900. (12 marks)

You may use the following in your answer:
- Cholera
- Public Health Acts

You **must** also use information of your own.

1796	Edward Jenner discovered the smallpox vaccine
1842	Edwin Chadwick published his *Report on the Sanitary Conditions of the Labouring Classes*
1847	Simpson discovered chloroform as an anaesthetic
1848	First Public Health Act
1852	Government made the smallpox vaccine compulsory
1854	Cholera epidemic
1854	John Snow proved that cholera was caused by dirty water
1858	The Great Stink
1859	Nightingale wrote *Notes on Nursing*
1861	Pasteur published his Germ Theory
1875	Second Public Health Act
1883	Koch discovered the microbe that caused cholera

Spot the mistakes

Below is a paragraph which is part of an answer to the question above. However, the paragraph has a series of factual mistakes. Once you have identified the mistakes, rewrite the paragraph.

In 1846 the British government passed the first Public Health Act. This was because the deadly disease typhoid returned to Britain. The government had listened to the advice from John Snow and passed an Act that would provide vaccinations to its citizens. Unfortunately, it had little impact because the measures were too expensive. When typhoid returned in 1854, Florence Nightingale was able to prove that it was spread by sour milk. But she was unable to explain how or why. In 1861, Robert Koch published his Germ Theory. He did this after experimenting with mice. The new understanding of the cause of disease and illness led to the government passing the second Public Health Act in 1865. This Act was compulsory and shows the change in attitudes towards the individual's role in public health.

c.1900–present: Medicine in modern Britain

The twentieth century saw great changes in medical diagnosis, treatment and prevention as a result of advancing science and technology. After accepting its responsibility for the health of the people, the government adopted a major role in providing medical care.

1 Ideas about the cause of disease and illness

REVISED

1.1 The influence of genetic factors on health

By 1900, it was clear to scientists that microbes did not cause all disease and illness. The causes of **hereditary diseases** were still unknown. The puzzle of hereditary diseases was solved in 1953 when **DNA** was discovered. It is now understood that Down's syndrome and cystic fibrosis are hereditary diseases.

The discovery of the human gene	Mapping of the human genome
In 1953, James Watson and Francis Crick saw the X-rays of DNA created by Rosalind Franklin and Maurice Wilkins Watson and Crick built their own model of DNA. Franklin corrected it and Wilkins shared clearer images with the team This helped Crick and Watson to understand the structure of DNA: that it was shaped as a double helix	Once the structure of DNA was understood, scientists were able to break it apart and look at the parts that caused hereditary diseases such as **haemophilia** The Human Genome Project began in 1990 and was completed in 2000. Scientists all over the world worked to decode and map the human **genome**. This map is used to look for mistakes in the human genome of people suffering from genetic conditions
Impact of the discovery	
The understanding of DNA has not led to the treatment of genetic conditions. However, it has given options to prevent diseases after the identification of particular genes. An example of this is breast cancer. Women can have their breasts removed if the gene linked to the disease is identified in their DNA in order to prevent them from possibly developing cancer	

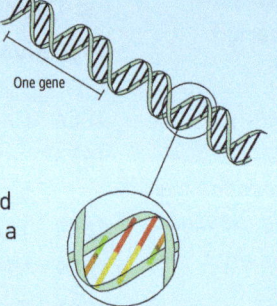

One gene

1.2 The influence of lifestyle factors on health

Our understanding of how lifestyle is linked to disease and illness has improved:

- Smoking is linked to a range of diseases including high blood pressure, cancers and heart disease.
- Diet has a huge impact on our health and we are advised to maintain a healthy food intake. For example, too much sugar can lead to type 2 diabetes and too much fat can lead to heart disease.
- Drinking too much alcohol can lead to liver disease and kidney problems.
- The sharing of bodily fluids, for example by having unprotected sex, can lead to the spread of certain diseases.
- Skin cancer can be caused by too much exposure to the sun without sunscreen.

> **Key terms**
>
> **DNA** Short for deoxyribonucleic acid. DNA carries genetic information about a living organism. DNA information determines characteristics such as hair and eye colour

> **Key terms**
>
> **Genome** The complete set of genes (DNA) in a particular organism. Every human being has unique DNA, unless they are identical twins
>
> **Haemophilia** A medical condition in which the ability of the blood to clot is severely reduced, causing the sufferer to bleed severely from even a slight injury
>
> **Hereditary diseases** Disease and illness caused by genetic factors and passed on from parents to their children

1.3 Improvements in diagnosis

The development of technology has enabled doctors to understand and diagnose illness and disease more quickly and accurately. Some examples include:

Technology	Description	Examples of use
X-ray	To see inside the human body without cutting it open	Diagnose broken bones
CT and MRI scans	Detailed imaging of internal organs	Diagnose internal damage, tumours and other growths
Ultrasound	A medical image produced from sound	Diagnose kidney stones, image an unborn baby
ECG	Electrocardiograms that measure heart activity	Measure irregular heart movement
Endoscope	A camera on the end of a thin tube used to see inside the body	Investigate digestive problems
Blood testing	Samples of blood are checked	Diagnose illness
Blood pressure monitor	Measures blood pressure	Diagnose high and low blood pressure

Key factor

Science and technology
The development of machines and computers since 1900 has improved diagnosis and allowed for more targeted treatment. Technology is advancing all of the time and so is the way that doctors diagnose disease and illness.

Revision task

Create a mind map of all of the ways that technology has advanced the diagnosis of illness since 1900.

Choosing a third cause

Below is an exam-style question. To answer it you need to explain three causes. It is sensible to make use of the two given points. However, you need to explain a third cause. In the spaces below the question, write down your choice and the reasons behind it.

Explain why there have been changes in understanding the causes of illness during the twentieth century.
(12 marks)

You may use the following in your answer:
- DNA
- Lifestyle

You **must** also use information of your own.

Reason: _____

Why I have chosen this reason: _____

Details to support this reason: _____

Complete the paragraph

Below is a paragraph which is part of an answer to the question in the 'Choosing a third cause' activity above. The paragraph gives a cause for change and some historical support but does not go on to develop the explanation.

1. Rewrite the paragraph with extra precise supporting knowledge and a full explanation linking back to the statement.
2. Complete the answer to this question.

> Understanding of the cause of illness has changed in the twentieth century as scientists and doctors have increased their understanding of the link between lifestyle and disease and illness. It is now accepted that smoking, diet, alcohol and tanning are the causes of disease. It is now accepted that smoking causes a variety of diseases, such as high blood pressure, a wide range of cancers and heart disease.

Edexcel GCSE (9–1) History Medicine in Britain

2 Approaches to prevention and treatment 1

2.1 Advances in medicines

The magic bullet

Magic bullet is used to describe a chemical cure that attacks microbes which cause a particular disease, without side-effects. For example:

- The first magic bullet, Salvarsan 606, was developed in 1909 by Paul Ehrlich as a treatment for syphilis.
- Gerhard Domagk followed in 1932 with the discovery of Prontosil. Prontosil was a cure for blood poisoning.

Antibiotics

In the early twentieth century, the first antibiotic was developed as a result of the development of penicillin.

2.2 Fleming, Florey and Chain's development of penicillin

Discovery	The development of penicillin revolutionised how infection was treated. Alexander Fleming, a British doctor, was researching substances that would cure simple infections. In 1928, Fleming noticed a mould on a dirty Petri dish that had killed the harmful staphylococcus bacteria that was growing in the dish. This mould was penicillin. Fleming published his findings in an article but did not pursue this any further
Development	In 1939, Howard Florey and Ernst Chain were researching antibiotics and they used Fleming's article. They grew their own penicillin mould and began experimenting
	In 1940, Florey and Chain tested penicillin on infected mice. The penicillin cured the infection
	In 1941, Florey and Chain had a human patient; a policeman who was suffering from blood poisoning. They began their experiment despite only having a small amount of penicillin. The policeman began to recover
	Because penicillin was difficult to make in large quantities they did not have enough to treat him for longer, and he died
	However, Florey and Chain had proven that penicillin could fight infection in a human
Mass production	Florey and Chain needed a factory that could mass produce penicillin and went to the USA for help. The US government funded 21 pharmaceutical companies to mass produce it. By D-Day, in June 1944, enough penicillin had been produced to treat all Allied casualties – over 2.3 million doses
Uses of penicillin and antibiotics	Penicillin is used to treat diseases caused by a certain family of bacteria. It is also used to prevent infection
	The development of other antibiotics followed and these are used daily to treat infections, such as streptomycin to treat tuberculosis and tetracycline to treat skin infections

2.3 High-tech medical and surgical treatment

The development of new machinery since 1900 has improved the treatment in hospitals. New high-tech medical and surgical treatments include:

- Radiotherapy and chemotherapy to target and shrink tumours growing inside the body.
- Dialysis to 'wash' the blood of patients with kidney failure.
- Prosthetic limbs to replace those lost, for example by soldiers in war.
- Transplant surgery, for example transplanting the kidneys, liver and heart.
- Keyhole surgery to prevent cutting into a patient's body.

> **Key terms**
>
> **Antibiotic** A medicine that destroys or limits the growth of bacteria in the human body
>
> **D-Day** The day (6 June 1944) in the Second World War on which Allied forces invaded northern France by means of beach landings in Normandy
>
> **Magic bullet** A chemical that kills certain bacteria without harming the body, for example Salvarsan 606 and Prontosil

> **Revision task**
>
> Create a timeline showing the main developments in the treatment of disease and illness since 1900.

Organising knowledge

Use the information on page 26 to complete the table below to show the factors that contributed to the development of penicillin in the twentieth century. First, cross out the factor(s) that did not contribute. Second, explain the role that each remaining factor played. For a reminder about each factor see page 5.

Individuals	
The Church	
The government	
Science and technology	
Attitudes in society	

Identify the view

Read the exam-style question below and identify the view that is offered about the development of penicillin in the early twentieth century.

'The main reason that penicillin was developed in the early twentieth century was because of the work of individuals.' How far do you agree? Explain your answer. (16 marks, with a further 4 marks available for spelling, punctuation and grammar.)

1 What view is offered by the statement about the development of penicillin?

_____

_____

2 How far do you agree? Use your knowledge to agree and disagree with the statement given in the question. To plan an answer to this question, complete the following table.

Knowledge which agrees with the statement	
Knowledge which disagrees with the statement	

3 Now write paragraphs that agree and disagree with the statement.

The statement is partially correct ...

The statement is partially incorrect ...

3 Approaches to prevention and treatment 2

REVISED

3.1 Change in care and treatment

The British government introduced the National Health Service (NHS) in 1948 to provide medical care for all people. It was the largest intervention by the government in medical care, and marked the end of its *laissez-faire* approach (see page 22).

With the NHS, the government aims to provide care for all people 'from the cradle to the grave' through:

- hospitals
- general practitioners (GPs)
- dentists
- ambulance services
- health visitors.

Throughout the 1960s, the British government made improvements to the NHS, such as:

- ensuring that hospitals were available across the whole of Britain
- giving GPs incentives to ensure they were up to date with medical developments.

3.2 New approaches to prevention

Mass vaccinations

The government introduced compulsory vaccinations throughout the twentieth century, including diphtheria in 1942 and polio in 1950. These vaccination campaigns were funded by the government to ensure that they were widespread.

Government legislation

The government has passed laws to ensure healthy living conditions. For example:

- The Clean Air Acts of 1956 and 1968 were passed to prevent **smog** caused by air pollution.
- As part of the Health Act of 2006, it was made illegal to smoke in all enclosed workplaces.

Government lifestyle campaigns

The government aims to help people prevent illness themselves through education and by promoting healthier lifestyles. Some examples of this are:

- advertising campaigns that warn against the dangers to health from binge drinking and drug use
- encouraging people to eat more healthily and get more exercise, such as the Change4Life campaign.

> **Exam tip**
>
> You need to be aware of how science and technology has improved all stages of the fight against lung cancer in the twenty-first century.

> **Key terms**
>
> **Bronchoscope** A fibre-optic cable that is passed into the windpipe in order to view the bronchi
>
> **General practitioner (GP)** A community-based doctor who treats minor illnesses. A GP will refer more serious cases of illness to a hospital
>
> **PET-CT scan** A CT scan creates a detailed picture of the inside of the body. A PET-CT scan is similar, but it contains a small amount of radioactive material that is injected instead of dye
>
> **Smog** A heavy fog caused by air pollution. Although smog is no longer a problem, the government continues to pass laws to protect people from air pollution

> **Key factors**
>
> **Science and technology** A range of scientific approaches and technology have been developed throughout the twentieth century that diagnose, prevent and treat disease and illness.
>
> **Government** Throughout the twentieth century, the government has taken a more active role in the prevention and treatment of disease and illness; more recently the focus has been on education and prevention.

3.3 The fight against lung cancer in the twenty-first century

Lung cancer is the second most common cancer in the UK and the number of deaths from this illness have risen throughout the twentieth century.

Diagnosis	By the time the disease is detected it is often too far advanced and so difficult to treat. Technology has enabled improvements. Doctors use a **PET-CT scan** or a dye to identify the cancerous cells. A **bronchoscope** can also be used to collect a sample of the cells
Treatment	If the cancer is detected early an operation to remove the tumour and the infected part of the lung can be carried out. Other treatments include: • transplants – cancerous cells can be replaced with those from a healthy donor • radiotherapy – waves of radiation are aimed at the tumour to shrink it • chemotherapy – patients are injected with different drugs to shrink the tumour before surgery to prevent the recurrence of cancer or to relieve the symptoms when surgery is not possible
Prevention	Evidence that cigarette smoking was linked to lung cancer was first published in 1950, but the government was slow to respond. As the death rate became too high to ignore, the government took the following action: • banned smoking in all public places in 2007, extended to cars carrying children in 2015 • raised the legal age for buying tobacco from 16 to 18 in 2007 • banned tobacco advertising in 1965, and banned cigarette advertising entirely in 2005 • removed cigarette products from display in shops in 2012 • introduced stop smoking campaigns and insisted on plain packaging Each year there is an increase in the taxation on tobacco products to encourage people to stop smoking

The comparison question

Look at the exam-style question below and the two answers. Which answer is better for comparing the key features of medical understanding? Why?

Explain one way in which the prevention of disease and illness was different in the nineteenth and twenty-first centuries. (4 marks)

ANSWER 1

In the nineteenth century, the British government took a *laissez-faire* approach to preventing disease and illness, believing it was not its responsibility. However, by the twenty-first century, the British government no longer had a *laissez-faire* approach to the health of its people and took action in preventing disease and illness by educating the people so that they could take control. This can be seen in the government-encouraged campaigns making the population aware of the dangers of smoking, binge drinking and drug use. It can also be seen in the Change4Life campaign.

ANSWER 2

In the nineteenth century, the British government did not take action preventing and treating disease and illness as it did not believe it was its responsibility. However, by the twenty-first century, the British government no longer had this approach and believed that it should educate the people so that they could take control. This can be seen in the government-encouraged campaigns making the population aware of the dangers of smoking, binge drinking and drug use.

Part 2 The British sector of the Western Front, 1914–18: injuries, treatment and the trenches

1 The context of the British sector of the Western Front

REVISED

Flanders and northern France

The Ypres Salient	The Somme
The scene of many battles during the First World War because it was on the way to the Channel ports of Calais and Dunkirk. The Germans wanted to capture these ports to cut off supplies to the British army	The Battle of the Somme lasted from July to November 1916 and took place along the River Somme
The **Ypres Salient** was vulnerable because the Germans had the advantageous position on higher ground. The German army could see the Allied movements and build stronger defences	It is remembered for its high casualty rate. On the first day of the battle the British army suffered nearly 60,000 casualties and 20,000 dead
Tunnelling and mines were used by the British at Hill 60, a man-made hill captured by the Germans, to regain control in April 1915	In total there were over 400,000 Allied casualties. This put enormous pressure on the medical services on the Western Front
The first Battle of Ypres took place between October and November 1914	
The second Battle of Ypres (April to May 1915) saw the first use of chlorine gas by the Germans	
The third Battle of Ypres took place in July to November 1917	
Arras	**Cambrai**
The Battle of Arras took place in April 1917	The Battle of Cambrai took place in October 1917
Before the battle, Allied soldiers had dug a network of tunnels below Arras. The tunnelling was made easy by the chalky ground. New tunnels joined with existing tunnels, caves and quarries. Rooms were created with running water and electricity. There was also a hospital (see page 34). These tunnels were used for safety and to allow troops to the front in secrecy	During this battle over 450 large-scale tanks were used by the Allies to launch a surprise assault on the German front line. Unfortunately, the tanks did not have enough infantry support. The British lost the ground they had taken

The trench system

The **trenches** dug in 1914 developed into an effective defensive network from 1915. The trenches were about 2.5 metres deep. They were dug in a zig-zag pattern and contained dugouts for men to take protective cover in when needed.

The front line	The trench nearest the enemy where the soldiers would shoot from
The command trench	10–20 metres behind the firing line
The support trench	200–500 metres behind the front line
The reserve trench	At least 100 metres behind the support trench. Reserve troops would be here ready to mount a counterattack if the enemy entered the front line
The communication trench	Linked the front line with the command, support and reserve trenches

Key terms

No Man's Land The land between the Allied and German trenches in the First World War

Trenches Long, narrow ditches dug during the First World War in which soldiers fought

Ypres Salient An area around Ypres in Belgium where many of the battles took place in the First World War

The impact of the terrain on helping the wounded

The trench system was complicated and made it hard to move the wounded from the trenches to the hospitals. This was because:

- It was difficult to move through the trench system because it contained equipment and men.
- Communication about the wounded was difficult, especially during major battles.
- It was hard to move around at night.
- Collecting the wounded from **No Man's Land** was dangerous because it was frequently done under fire.
- No Man's Land and the trenches were often deep in mud, which made movement difficult.
- Stretcher bearers found it difficult to move around the corners.
- Transport of the wounded was difficult because of these conditions (see page 34).

Revision task
Draw and label your own copy of the trench system.

Exam tip
You need to be able to explain the impact that the terrain of the Western Front had on the care and treatment of the wounded.

Eliminate irrelevance

Here is an exam-style question:

Describe two features of the trench system on the Western Front. (4 marks)

Below is an answer to this question. Read the answer and identify parts that are not relevant to the question. Draw a line through the information that is irrelevant and justify your deletions in the margin.

> The trench system used in the First World War by the British began in 1914 and was improved from 1915. The trenches were dug quickly and so were very simple to start with. There was the front line trench, which was closest to the enemy and is where soldiers would fire and mount an attack from. Behind the front line trench was the command trench. The reserve line trench was the furthest away from the front line. It was here that soldiers would be mobilised from for a counterattack should the enemy make it into the front line trenches. Between the British and German trenches was an area of unoccupied land called No Man's Land.

2 Conditions requiring treatment on the Western Front

Ill health

Complaint	Cause	Symptoms	Treatment and prevention	Impact
Trench fever	Transmitted by body lice	Flu-like symptoms; high temperature, severe headaches, shivering and aching muscles	**Treatment:** drugs were trialled, such as quinine and Salvarsan, but without success. Passing an electric current through the affected area was used effectively **Prevention:** by 1918, the cause had been identified as lice: • clothes were disinfected with repellent gel • delousing stations were set up	Affected nearly half a million men on the Western Front
Trench foot	Soldiers stood in the mud and waterlogged trenches, which caused painful swelling in their feet	Tight boots added to the problem because they restricted the blood flow. Later, **gangrene** would set in	**Treatment:** soldiers were advised to clean and dry their feet. In the worst cases, amputation **Prevention:** • changing socks and keeping feet dry • rubbing whale oil into feet to protect them	During the winter of 1914 and 1915, over 20,000 Allied men were affected
Shell-shock	Stressful conditions of war	Tiredness, nightmares, headaches, uncontrollable shaking and a mental breakdown	The condition was not well understood during the war **Treatment:** • mainly consisted of rest • some soldiers received treatment back in Britain	It is estimated that 80,000 British troops experienced shell-shock. Some men were accused of cowardice. Punishments for this included being shot

Weapons of war

- *Rifles*: loaded from a cartridge case which created automatic rapid fire, rather than one bullet at a time. Bullets were pointed so that they drove deeper into the body.
- *Machine guns*: had more speed than rifles and could fire 500 rounds a minute. They devastated attacking forces advancing over No Man's Land. Bullets, from machine guns and rifles, would pierce organs and fracture bones.
- *Artillery*: throughout the war, cannons grew bigger and became more powerful, such as the British howitzer which could send 900-kilogram shells. Bombardments were continuous and in some cases lasted weeks and months. Artillery fire caused half of all casualties.
- *Shrapnel*: **shrapnel** caused maximum damage as it exploded mid-air above the enemy. It was most effective against troops advancing across No Man's Land, while shells targeted soldiers in the trenches. An exploded shell or shrapnel could immediately kill or injure a soldier. Together these were responsible for 58 per cent of wounds. In most cases, shrapnel injured the arms and legs of soldiers.

Soldiers experienced an increased number of head injuries as a result of all of the above weapons. In 1915, a steel helmet replaced the soft caps of soldiers. In a trial, it was estimated that the helmet reduced fatal head injuries by 80 per cent.

Key terms

Gangrene When body tissue decomposes due to a loss of blood supply

Shrapnel A hollow shell that was filled with steel balls or lead, together with gunpowder and a timer fuse

Revision task

Summarise the weapons and wounds of war:
- rifles
- machine guns
- artillery
- shrapnel.

Gas attacks

Chlorine	Phosgene	Mustard
First used by Germans in 1915	First used by Germans in 1915	First used by Germans in 1917
Led to death by suffocation	Faster acting than chlorine, but with similar effects	An odourless gas that worked in 12 hours
In July 1915, gas masks were given to all British troops. Before this soldiers would urinate on handkerchiefs and hold these to their faces to prevent the gas getting into their lungs	Could kill an exposed person within two days	Caused blisters and could burn the skin through clothing

It was hard to target a particular place with gas and so it was not used regularly as a weapon in the First World War. Gas was the cause of fewer than five per cent of British deaths. The effects of gas attacks – blindness, loss of taste and smell and coughing – only lasted for a few weeks. Sufferers were given oxygen and had their skin cleansed.

Exam tip

You need to be able to make links between the nature of fighting in the First World War and the illnesses that soldiers suffered from.

You're the examiner

Below is an exam-style question.

Describe two features of the gas attacks on the Western Front. (4 marks)

1. Below are a mark scheme and an answer to this question. Read the answer and the mark scheme. Decide how many marks it would get. Write the mark along with a justification for your choice below.

Mark scheme

Award 1 mark for each valid feature identified up to a maximum of two features. The second mark should be awarded for supporting information.

STUDENT ANSWER

Chlorine gas was used in the Western Front by the Germans in 1915. Chlorine gas led to death by suffocation after attacking a victim's lungs.

Mark [ ]   Reason _____

2. Now suggest what the student has to do to achieve more marks.
3. Write an answer that would achieve more marks.

3 Helping the wounded on the Western Front

The evacuation route

Survival depended on the speed of treatment and so the aim was to treat all soldiers quickly.

Stage 1	Stretcher bearers	Stretcher bearers would advance on No Man's Land at night or during a break in fighting to collect the dead and wounded. Each battalion had sixteen stretcher bearers and it took four men to carry a stretcher
Stage 2	Regimental Aid Post (RAP)	The RAP was always close to the front line. The battalion regimental medical officer was in the RAP. He identified those who were lightly wounded and those soldiers who needed more medical attention
Stage 3	Field Ambulance and Dressing Station	A Field Ambulance was a large mobile medical unit with medical officers, support staff and, from 1915, some nurses. The Dressing Station was where emergency treatment was given to the wounded. They were about a mile behind the front line. Here a system of triage was set up, where the more and less seriously wounded were separated
Stage 4	Casualty Clearing Station (CCS)	The CCS was the first large well-equipped medical unit that the wounded would experience. The CCS contained X-ray machines and wards with beds. They were located in tents or huts about ten miles from the fighting
Stage 5	Base Hospitals	The Base Hospital was usually a civilian hospital or a converted building. Soldiers would arrive by train, motor ambulance or by canal because the journey was less uncomfortable. They had operating theatres, X-ray departments and specialist areas for gas poisoning. From the Base Hospital, most patients were sent back to Britain in hospital trains, which had been converted

Soldiers received better care as the war progressed. In 1914, there were no motor ambulances, and the horse-drawn ambulances were unable to cope with the great number of casualties. By November 1915, there were 250 motor ambulances in France. Ambulance trains were also introduced to carry up to 800 casualties. Ambulance barges were also used to carry the wounded along the River Somme.

The underground hospital at Arras

During the Battle of Arras, 160,000 soldiers were killed; and over 7000 were wounded in the first three days. Despite this, the evacuation route here worked well. In 1916, the existing tunnels and quarries were extended. They created an underground town for soldiers to live in with running water and electricity. This location also included a hospital with 700 beds and operating theatres.

RAMC

All medical officers belonged to the RAMC. The membership increased from 9000 in 1914 to 113,000 in 1918 as the number of wounded grew. Doctors had to learn quickly about conditions and wounds they had never faced before.

FANY

Initially the nurses on the front line were the well-trained Queen Alexandra's nurses. The government turned away volunteer nurses. However, this attitude changed as the number of casualties increased. The work of volunteers involved professional nursing in operating theatres to scrubbing floors. Women of the FANY helped the wounded as ambulance drivers and nurses once the British army changed their policy towards volunteers in 1916. FANY units also carried supplies to the front and drove motorised kitchens to supply food.

Key terms

FANY First Aid Nursing Yeomanry. Founded in 1907 by a soldier who hoped they would be a nursing cavalry to help the wounded in battle

RAMC Royal Army Medical Corps. This organisation organised and provided medical care. It consisted of all ranks from doctors to ambulance drivers and stretcher bearers

Triage A system of splitting the wounded into groups according to who needed the most urgent attention

Revision task

Summarise the part played in treatment of the wounded by the following: stretcher bearers, horse-drawn and motor ambulances, train and canal ambulances.

The utility question

Look at the two sources, the exam-style question and the two answers below. Which answer is the best answer to the question and why? You could look at page 42 for guidance on how to answer the utility question to help you make your judgement.

SOURCE A

Stretcher bearers removing a wounded officer.

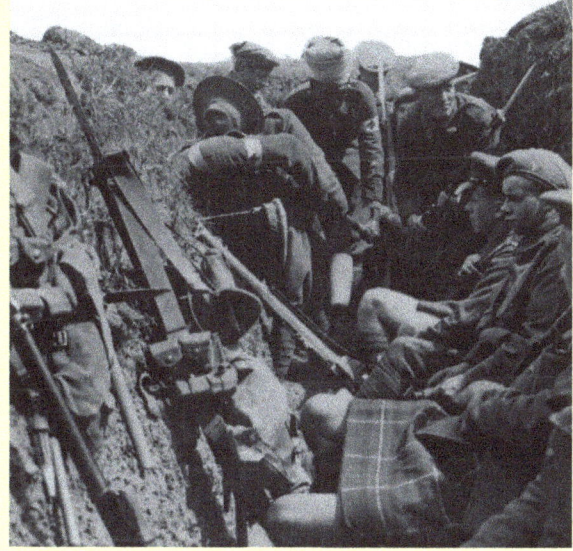

SOURCE B

An extract from an article in the Journal of the Royal Army Medical Corps, 1915.

Admirable as was the organisation of the large base hospitals, the transport of the wounded from the fighting line seems to have been very badly managed during the advance of the Germans through Belgium and northern France. The supply of motor ambulances proved totally inadequate and the slightly wounded had to shift for themselves and squeeze into goods trains.

How useful are Sources A and B for an enquiry into the problems that faced those helping the wounded on the Western Front? (8 marks)

ANSWER 1

Source A is useful for this enquiry because it shows the stretcher bearers in the First World War having to walk with the wounded through narrow and crowded trenches. Source B is useful for the same enquiry because it tells us that there were not enough motor ambulances and so the wounded had to squeeze into trains.

ANSWER 2

Source A is useful for an enquiry into the problems faced in helping the wounded during the First World War because it shows the stretcher bearers in the First World War having to walk with the wounded through narrow and crowded trenches. From my own knowledge, I know that the stretcher bearers would also have had to collect the wounded from No Man's Land during a break in fighting or at night. This caused problems because they were unable to see the wounded soldiers. The stretcher bearer would have to carry the wounded across shell-craters, which was also dangerous because they were difficult to see, and avoid, at night. Source B is useful for the same enquiry because it tells us that there were not enough motor ambulances and so the wounded had to squeeze into trains. From my own knowledge, I know that trains were converted into hospitals and used to transport the wounded back to Britain, as well as canal boats.

Which answer is better?
_____

Why?
_____

4 The impact of the Western Front on medicine and surgery 1

Treating wounds and infection

By 1900, most operations were carried out using aseptic methods, but it was not possible to carry out aseptic surgery (see page 20) on the Western Front because treatment needed to be portable. This led to problems treating infections caused by **gas gangrene**, and other treatments had to be found.

- Wound incision or **debridement** – this needed to be done quickly and the wound closed to prevent the spread of infection.
- The Carrel–Dakin method – this involved using a sterilised salt solution in the wound through a tube. However, the solution only lasted six hours and so had to be made as it was needed, which was difficult at times of high demand.
- Amputation – if neither of the above had worked, the only option left to surgeons was to remove the wounded limb. By 1918, 240,000 men had lost limbs.

The Thomas splint

Men with a gunshot or shrapnel wound only had a twenty per cent chance of survival in 1915. This was because the wounds created a **compound fracture**. This was particularly dangerous when the thigh bone (femur) was fractured because it damaged the muscle and caused major bleeding into the thigh.

The splint that was being used to transport wounded men did not keep the leg rigid. From 1916, the Thomas splint was used, which stopped two joints moving and increased the survival rate from this type of wound to 82 per cent.

X-rays

In 1895, William Röntgen, a German physicist, discovered X-rays. From 1896, **radiology departments** were opening in a number of hospitals. British hospitals applied X-rays to a medical setting. X-rays enabled a surgeon to carry out a diagnosis before an operation took place and would prove useful on the Western Front.

X-rays were used from the start of the war to locate bullets and shrapnel. These needed to be removed from wounds to prevent infection. Overall, the use of X-rays was success. However, there were some problems:

- X-rays could not detect all objects in the body. Some items, such as clothing, went unnoticed until doctors looked for them during the operation.
- A wounded soldier had to remain still for several minutes for an X-ray to be taken.
- The tubes used in an X-ray were fragile and overheated quickly. This meant that X-ray machines could only be used for an hour and then had to be left to cool down. During an offensive this was a major problem. The solution was to use three machines in rotation.

The use of mobile X-ray units

There were six **mobile X-ray units** operating in the British sector of the Western Front. These were used to locate shrapnel and bullet wounds. They were transported around the Western Front in a truck, enabling more soldiers to be treated quickly. The mobile X-ray unit could go to the location of a battle, rather than wait for soldiers to be transported. The quality of X-rays taken by the mobile units was not as good, but proved sufficient to locate bullets and shrapnel.

> **Key terms**
>
> **Compound fracture** An injury where the broken bone pierces the skin and increases the risk of infection
>
> **Debridement** The cutting away of dead, damaged and infected tissue around the wound
>
> **Gas gangrene** An infection that produces gas in gangrenous wounds. Infection was more likely as the soldiers' wounds were exposed to soil containing fertiliser
>
> **Mobile X-ray unit** A portable X-ray unit that could be moved around the Western Front in a truck
>
> **Radiology department** The hospital department where X-rays are carried out

> **Revision task**
>
> Summarise the following developments in surgery during the First World War:
> - treating infection
> - the Thomas splint
> - mobile X-ray units.

Complete the answer

Below is an exam-style question and an answer to this question. The answer identifies two features, but does not develop them with any supporting knowledge. Annotate the answer to complete it by adding the support.

Describe two features of the treatment of wounds on the Western Front. (4 marks)

> The Thomas splint was used in surgery on the Western Front. Mobile X-ray units were also used on the Western Front.

The utility question

Look at the two sources, the exam-style question and the two answers below. Which answer is the best answer to the question and why? You could look at page 42 for guidance on how to answer the utility question to help you make your judgement.

How useful are Sources A and B for an enquiry into surgery and the treatment of wounds on the Western Front? (8 marks)

SOURCE B

French medics locating a bullet with an X-ray machine at a French field hospital during the First World War.

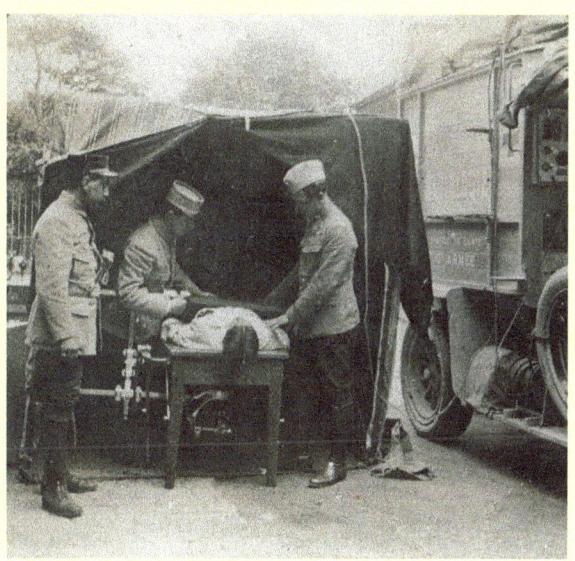

SOURCE A

From 'A report on Gas Gangrene' by Anthony Bowlby, Consulting Surgeon to the British Army, October 1914.

The gangrene found amongst our wounded soldiers is directly due to infection introduced at the time of the wound, and this is likely to occur if muddy clothing has been carried by the projectile, or if earth has been carried by the explosion.

ANSWER 1

> Source A is useful for an enquiry into surgery and the treatment of wounds on the Western Front because it tells us about gas gangrene and how it was caused by an infected wound. From my own knowledge, I know that this problem was made worse during the First World War because many soldiers' wounds were exposed to soil that was full of fertiliser.

ANSWER 2

> Source A is useful for an enquiry into surgery and the treatment of wounds on the Western Front because it is from an official contemporary report published in October 1914 by Anthony Bowlby, a consulting surgeon. Bowlby would have seen first-hand the conditions on the Western Front facing the surgeons and had experience in the number of soldiers whose wounds developed gas gangrene. From my own knowledge, I know that this problem was made worse during the First World War because many soldiers' wounds were exposed to soil that was full of fertiliser.

5 The impact of the Western Front on medicine and surgery 2

REVISED

The development of blood transfusions and the storage of blood

Blood loss was a major problem in surgery before the twentieth century. The first experiments in **blood transfusion** were performed in 1819 by James Blundell. As blood could not be stored, it had to be used as soon as possible. Transfusions were carried out with the donor (the person giving the blood) being directly connected by a tube to the recipient (the person receiving the blood).

There were problems with the early use of blood transfusions:

- Blood clots as soon as it leaves the body and so the tube became blocked up.
- The blood of the donor was sometimes rejected by the recipient because they were not compatible. Blood groups were discovered by Karl Landsteiner in 1901.
- There was a danger of infection from unsterilised equipment. However, this problem was being solved with the introduction of aseptic surgery.

Blood transfusions were used at Base Hospitals by the British on the Western Front from 1915. A syringe and tube were used to transfer the donor blood to the patient. This was extended to Casualty Clearing Stations from 1917. A portable blood transfusion kit was used close to the front line, designed by a doctor called Geoffrey Keynes.

> **Key terms**
>
> **Blood transfusion** Blood taken from a healthy person and given to another person
>
> **General anaesthetic** Putting a patient to sleep during an operation
>
> **Local anaesthetic** The area being operated was numbed to prevent pain, but the patient remained awake during the operation

The blood bank at Cambrai

- In 1915, it was discovered that by adding sodium citrate to blood the need for donor-to-recipient transfusion was removed as blood could be stored and clotting prevented.
- In 1916, it was discovered that adding a citrate glucose solution to blood allowed it to be stored for up to four weeks.

Stored blood was used at the Battle of Cambrai in 1917. Blood was stored in glass bottles at a blood bank and used to treat badly wounded soldiers throughout the battle.

Other new techniques in the treatment of wounds

- *Brain surgery*: new techniques for dealing with brain injuries were developed for the Western Front that included using a magnet to remove metal fragments from the brain. A **local anaesthetic** was used in operations rather than a **general anaesthetic**. This prevented the brain from swelling and decreased the risks in an operation.
- *Plastic surgery*: a New Zealand doctor, Harold Gillies, was sent to the Western Front in 1915. Gillies became interested in facial reconstruction – replacing and restoring parts of the face that had been destroyed by the weapons of war. Skin grafts were developed, where skin was taken from another part of the patient's body and used to repair the wound.

Organising knowledge

Study the advances in surgery during the First World War on pages 36 and 38. Make a copy of the table below. Complete it to show the progress made as a result of the war.

Factor	Before First World War	During First World War
War wounds		
Infection		
X-rays		
Blood transfusions		
Plastic surgery		

Organising knowledge

Study the different types of sources available to a historian when enquiring into the Western Front in the table below. Complete the table. For each type of source explain what aspects of injuries, treatment and the trenches covered in this book it would be useful for and explain the advantages of using it. For example, hospital records would be useful in providing the number of soldiers treated during an offensive. This information would not have been produced for propaganda and so would give the historian reliable, accurate figures.

Types of sources	Useful for …	Advantages
National army records for individual soldiers		
National newspaper reports		
Government reports on aspects of the war		
Medical articles by doctors and nurses who took part in the war		
Personal accounts of medical treatments by soldiers, doctors, nurses or others who were involved		
Photographs		
Hospital records		
Army statistics		

Edexcel GCSE (9–1) History Medicine in Britain

Exam focus

Your History GCSE is made up of three exams:

- For Paper 1 you have one hour and 15 minutes to answer questions on a thematic study and historic environment, in your case Medicine through time, c1250–present and The British sector of the Western Front, 1914–18: injuries, treatments and the trenches.
- In Paper 2 you have one hour and 45 minutes to answer questions on a period study and a British depth study.
- In Paper 3 you have one hour and 20 minutes to answer questions on a modern depth study.

For Paper 1 you have to answer the following types of questions. Each requires you to demonstrate different historical skills:

- **Question 1** is a key features question in which you have to describe two features and characteristics of the period.
- **Question 2** includes two sub-questions on a source enquiry which test your source analysis skills as well as your ability to frame a historical question.
- **Question 3** is a key features question in which you have to describe the similarity or difference in medicine between two time periods.
- **Question 4** is a causation question which asks you to explain why something happened.
- **Questions 5 and 6** are analytical questions that ask you to evaluate change, continuity and significance in medicine.

The table below gives a summary of the question types for Paper 1 and what you need to do.

Question number	Marks	Key words	You need to ...
1	4	Describe two features of ...	• Identify two features • Add supporting information for each feature
2(a)	8	How useful are Sources A and B for an enquiry into ... ? Explain your answer, using Sources A and B and your knowledge of the historical context	• Ensure that you explain the value of the contents of each of the sources • Explain how the provenance of each source affects the value of the contents • You need to support your answer with your knowledge of the given topic
2(b)	4	How could you follow up Source B to find out more about ... In your answer you must give the question you would ask and the type of source you could use	• Select a detail from Source B that could form the basis of a follow-up enquiry • Write a question that is linked to this detail and enquiry • Identify an appropriate source for the enquiry • Explain how the source might help answer your follow-up question
3	4	Explain one way in which ... were similar/different in the ... and ... centuries	• Identify a similarity or difference • Support the comparison with specific detail from both periods
4	12	Explain why ... You may use the following in your answer: [two given points]. You **must** also use information of your own	• Explain at least three causes – you can use the points in the question but must also use at least one point of your own • Ensure that you focus the causes on the question
5/6	20	'Statement'. How far do you agree? Explain your answer. You may use the following in your answer: [two given points]. You **must** also use information of your own	• Ensure you agree and disagree with the statement • Use the given points and your own knowledge • Ensure you write a conclusion giving your final judgement on the question • There are up to 4 marks for spelling, punctuation, grammar and the use of specialist terminology

Question 1: Key features

Below is an example of a key features question which is worth 4 marks.

Describe two features of the weapons used on the Western Front.

Feature 1: _____

_____

Feature 2: _____

_____

How to answer

You have to identify two features and add supporting information for each. For each of the two features you are given space to write. Remember you need to identify **two** different features.

Below is a sample answer to this key features question with comments around it.

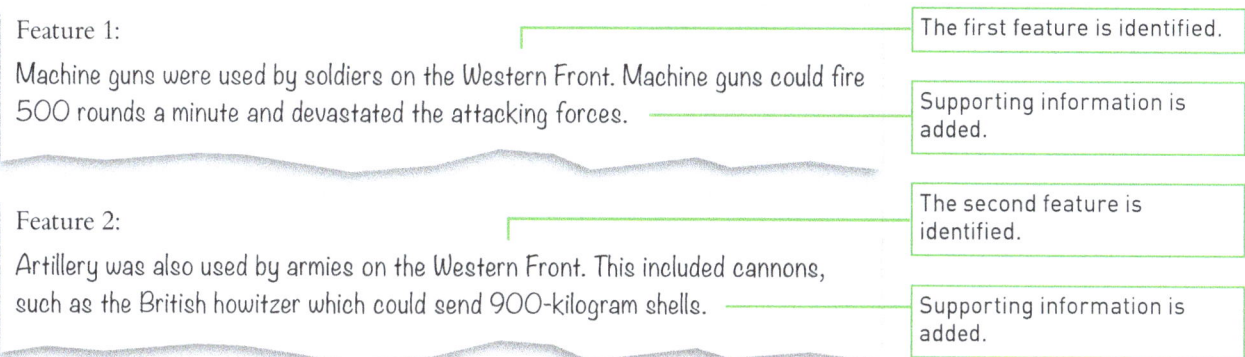

Feature 1:
Machine guns were used by soldiers on the Western Front. Machine guns could fire 500 rounds a minute and devastated the attacking forces.

- The first feature is identified.
- Supporting information is added.

Feature 2:
Artillery was also used by armies on the Western Front. This included cannons, such as the British howitzer which could send 900-kilogram shells.

- The second feature is identified.
- Supporting information is added.

Complete the answer

Describe two features of the evacuation route on the Western Front.

Here is the first part of an answer to this question.

Feature 1:

> The wounded were first collected by a stretcher bearer. Each battalion had sixteen stretcher bearers and it took four men to carry a stretcher.

1. Highlight the following:
   - Where the feature has been identified.
   - Where supporting information has been added.
2. Now add a second feature.

   Feature 2: _____

   _____

Question 2: Source analysis

Question 2 is divided into two parts.

- Question 2(a) is a utility question on two sources. You have to explain how useful each source is to a historical enquiry.
- Question 2(b) is an analysis question that asks you to use sources – you have to explain a follow-up enquiry and the source that you would use.

Question 2(a): Utility

Below is an example of a utility question which is worth 8 marks. The sources will be labelled Source A and Source B.

Study Sources A and B. How useful are Sources A and B for an enquiry into the impact of the terrain on the transport of the wounded on the Western Front? Explain your answer, using Sources A and B and your own knowledge of the historical context. (8 marks)

SOURCE A

No Man's Land on the Western Front, 1917.

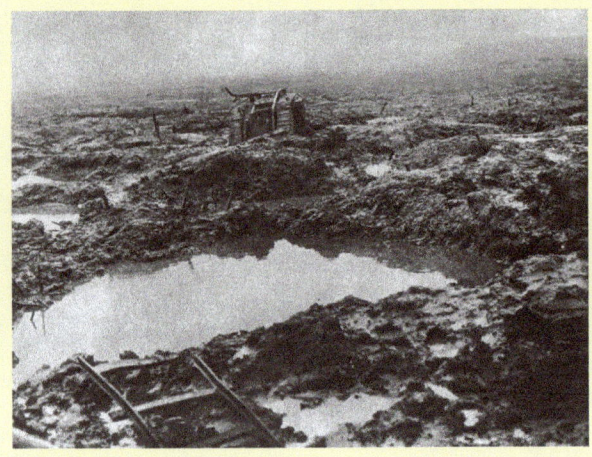

SOURCE B

From the recorded memories of William Easton, East Anglian Field Ambulance. He was eighteen years old in 1916. Here he described conditions near Ypres in 1917.

Up at Ypres we used to go up the line and we'd be waist deep in mud. We were carrying the wounded down near a place called Hooge, where had been a terrible amount of fighting. One trip down a trench in those conditions and you would all be all in – exhausted. If you got two or three wounded men down in a day, that was all you could expect to do. We had to carry men in fours there and we had to be very careful because you could do more damage to a man than the shell if you jolted him too much or he fell off the stretcher. To make carrying easier we had slings which we put round our shoulders and over the stretcher's handles.

How to answer

- Explain the value and limitations of the contents of each source and try to add some contextual knowledge when you make a point.
- Explain the value and limitations of the provenance of each source and try to add some contextual knowledge when you make a point.
- In your conclusion give a final judgement on the relative value of each source. For example, one source might provide one view of an event, the other source a different view.

Key term

Provenance Who wrote or created the source, when, and for what purpose. This can have a big impact on what the source tells us.

Below is part of a sample Level 3 answer to this question in which is explained the utility of Source A. Read it and the comments around it.

> Source A is useful because it suggests that the shell holes throughout No Man's Land caused an obstacle to the stretcher bearers who were collecting the dead and wounded. This was the case because stretcher bearers would often go into No Man's Land at night or during a break in the fighting. At these times it would have been difficult for them to see the shell holes. The usefulness of Source A is further enhanced by its provenance. It is a photograph taken in 1917 and so it shows exactly what No Man's Land would have looked like at this point in time and could not have been altered. However, a historian must be careful because it may not be typical of No Man's Land throughout the Western Front and may not have looked the same at all locations along the line of the trenches.

- A judgement is made on the value of the content of the source.
- Own knowledge is used to support this judgement.
- The provenance of the source is taken into account when making a judgement on its utility.

Analysing provenance

Now write your own Level 3 answer on Source B. Remember to take into account how the provenance affects the usefulness of the source content.

Quick quizzes at www.hoddereducation.co.uk/myrevisionnotes

Question 2(b): Framing a historical question

Below is an example of a source question requiring you to frame an enquiry. This is worth 4 marks.

How could you follow up Source B to find out more about the impact of the terrain on the transport of the wounded on the Western Front? In your answer, you must give the question you would ask and the type of source you could use.

How to answer

You have to identify a follow-up enquiry and explain how you would carry this out. For each of the questions you are given space to write. Below is a sample answer to this question with comments around it.

Detail in Source B that I would follow up:
I would follow up on what Easton says about the further damage that stretcher bearers and the conditions could cause wounded men.

The follow-up enquiry is identified.

Question I would ask:
What wounds were made worse by jolts whilst on the stretcher?

The linked question is asked.

What type of source I could use:
Hospital records.

An appropriate source is identified.

How this might help answer my question:
Hospital records could detail the nature of wounds that soldiers arrived with and whether they were caused by the fighting or the conditions while on the stretcher.

An explanation of how the source would help with the follow-up enquiry.

Question 3: Similarity or difference

Below is an example of a key features question which is worth 4 marks.

Explain one way in which understanding of the causes of illness was different in the late nineteenth and twentieth centuries.

How to answer

- Explain the difference between the two time periods.
- Use specific information from both time periods to support the comparison, showing good knowledge and understanding.

Below is a sample answer to this with comments around it.

In the late nineteenth century, disease and illness was explained by germs. Louis Pasteur had published his Germ Theory in 1861 to prove this. His theory was further developed by Robert Koch, who went on to identify the specific bacteria that caused tuberculosis and anthrax. However, by the twenty-first century it was also understood that disease could also be hereditary and not caused by bacteria. DNA was discovered in 1953 by Crick and Watson. Since DNA was first discovered, scientists have been able to show that specific genes pass on disease such as Down's syndrome and cystic fibrosis.

The belief about the cause of disease in the nineteenth century is identified.

Own knowledge is used to support this.

The change in belief about the cause of disease in the twentieth century is identified.

Own knowledge is used to support this.

Exam focus

Develop the detail

Below is a question and part of an answer. Read the answer and develop the detail.

Explain one way in which ideas about the cause of disease were different in the seventeenth and nineteenth centuries.

> In the seventeenth century it was believed that miasma (bad air) was the cause of disease. However, by the nineteenth century scientists had discovered that germs were the cause of disease.

Question 4: Causation

Below is an example of a causation question which is worth 12 marks.

Explain why there was so much opposition to Jenner's vaccination against smallpox.

You may use the following in your answer.
- Inoculation
- The Royal Society

You **must** also include information of your own.

How to answer

- You need to explain at least three causes. This could be the two mentioned in the question and one of your own. You don't have to use the points given in the question, you could decide to make more points of your own instead.
- You need to fully explain each cause and support your explanation with precise knowledge, ensuring that each cause is fully focused on the question.

Below is part of an answer to the question.

> There was a lot of opposition to Jenner's smallpox vaccination at the beginning of the nineteenth century. Doctors were used to giving inoculations and did not want to change their approach. The Royal Society did not help when they said that Jenner's idea was too revolutionary and refused to publish his book. The Anti-Vaccine Society was set up to oppose the vaccination. They did this by publishing cartoons that made fun of the vaccine and tried to scare people into not trusting and therefore not having the vaccination. One such cartoon showed people who had the vaccine turning into cows. Many religious believers thought it was against God's law to give people an animal disease.

- Opposition is described. However, there is no explicit focus on the question.
- The supporting evidence is not precise enough.
- The answer is losing focus on the question.

Make an improvement

Try improving the answer. An example of a better answer to this question is on page 45 for you to check your own answer against.

Your point is a short answer to the question. You then back this up with lots of examples to demonstrate all the knowledge you have learned during your studies: this is the section that proves you have studied and revised, rather than just guessing. Finally, you will link that knowledge to the question by explaining it in a final sentence.

- Point: passing my GCSE History exam will be very helpful in the future.
- Example: for example, it will help me to continue my studies next year.
- Explain: this will help me to get the job I want in the future.

Exam tip

Writing a good paragraph to explain an answer to something is as easy as PEEing: Point, Example, Explain.

44 Quick quizzes at www.hoddereducation.co.uk/myrevisionnotes

Below is a sample Level 4 answer to the causation question on page 44 with comments around it.

There was a lot of opposition to Jenner's smallpox vaccination at the beginning of the nineteenth century. One cause of the opposition was a lack of acceptance from the medical profession. Doctors were used to giving inoculations and did not want to change their approach. The Royal Society did not help when they said that Jenner's idea was too revolutionary and refused to publish his book.

The first cause is introduced and immediately focuses on the question.

The supporting evidence is precise and relevant to the question.

There was also opposition from the religious community. The Anti-Vaccine Society was set up to oppose the vaccination. They did this by publishing cartoons that made fun of the vaccine and tried to scare people into not trusting and therefore not having the vaccination. One such cartoon showed people who had the vaccine turning into cows. The Anti-Vaccine Society was set up in 1866. Many religious believers thought it was against God's law to give people an animal disease. It was believed that smallpox was sent as a punishment for sin and that only prayer and living a godly life could cure the disease.

The second cause is introduced and linked to the first cause and immediately focuses on the question.

The supporting evidence is precise and relevant to the question.

Jenner's inability to explain how his smallpox vaccine worked did not help to reduce the opposition. Pasteur did not publish his Germ Theory until 1861, so Jenner did not know that bacteria caused disease. This meant that he did not know exactly how vaccination worked and Jenner wasn't able to explain it to others. The longer term consequence of this was that it was not possible to learn from this discovery how to prevent the spread of other diseases. Without a clear explanation, the opposition to the smallpox vaccine continued.

The third cause is introduced and linked to the second cause and immediately focuses on the question. Notice that this is a cause not mentioned in the question.

The supporting evidence is precise and relevant to the question.

Now have a go

Explain why some changes took place in medical knowledge during the period c.1500–c.1700.

You may use the following in your answer:
- The Royal Society
- Vesalius

You **must** also use information of your own.

Question 5 and 6: A judgement about change, continuity and significance

Below is an example of question 5 and 6, which asks you to make a judgement about how far you agree with the statement. It is worth 20 marks (4 of these are for spelling, punctuation, grammar and the use of specialist terminology).

You may use the following in your answer.
- 1848 Public Health Act
- John Snow

You **must** also include information of your own.

'Edwin Chadwick's Report was the main reason why public health in towns improved during the nineteenth century.' Do you agree? Explain your answer.

How to answer

You need to give a balanced answer which agrees and disagrees with the statement using evidence from the bullet points as well as your own knowledge. Here is one way you could approach this:

- agree with the view with evidence from a bullet point and your own knowledge
- disagree with the view with evidence, possibly from the other bullet point and your own knowledge
- agree/disagree with the view (depending on statement) with another point from your own knowledge
- make a final judgement on whether you agree or disagree with the statement.

Below is part of an answer to this question which agrees with the view given in the statement.

> The public health in towns did improve during the nineteenth century and one reason for this was due to Edwin Chadwick's report. In 1842, Edwin Chadwick wrote his 'Report on the Sanitary Conditions of the Labouring Classes'. In this report, Chadwick showed that the poor lived in dirty, overcrowded conditions which caused a huge amount of illness. Due to this, many people were too sick to work and so became poorer still. This had an effect on the richer people because they had to pay more taxes to help the poor. Chadwick suggested that taxes should be cut and money should be saved in the long run by improving drainage and sewers, removing refuse from streets and houses, providing clean water supplies and appointing medical officers in each area to check on these reforms. Initially, there was opposition to Chadwick's ideas due to the initial need to increase taxes and for the government to get involved in local matters. However, after an outbreak of cholera in 1848, the government passed the 1848 Public Health Act which led to many towns improving their public health. This shows that Chadwick was important because he pushed the government to act in 1848 for the first time.

- The answer immediately focuses on the question.
- Support is provided from own knowledge.
- Explanation is provided using the first bullet point.

Now have a go

1. Have a go at another paragraph by disagreeing with the view given in the statement and using the second bullet point.
2. Write another paragraph that disagrees or agrees with the statement using another point from your own knowledge.
3. Write a conclusion giving your final judgement on the question.